100 Challenges in Cardiology

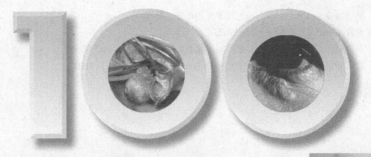

100
Challenges
in Cardiology

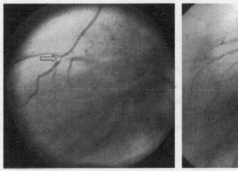
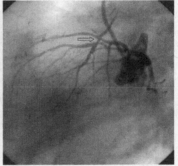

David R Ramsdale
Simon Modi
The Liverpool Heart and Chest Hospital, Liverpool, UK

World Scientific

NEW JERSEY · LONDON · SINGAPORE · BEIJING · SHANGHAI · HONG KONG · TAIPEI · CHENNAI

Published by

World Scientific Publishing Co. Pte. Ltd.
5 Toh Tuck Link, Singapore 596224
USA office: 27 Warren Street, Suite 401-402, Hackensack, NJ 07601
UK office: 57 Shelton Street, Covent Garden, London WC2H 9HE

British Library Cataloguing-in-Publication Data
A catalogue record for this book is available from the British Library.

ISBN-13 978-981-4307-14-7 (pbk)
ISBN-10 981-4307-14-9 (pbk)

Typeset by Stallion Press
Email: enquiries@stallionpress.com

Printed in Singapore.

To our wives, Bernie and Jenny
May the Force be with them!

David R Ramsdale BSc, MB ChB, MD, FRCP is Consultant Cardiologist at The Liverpool Heart and Chest Hospital, Liverpool, UK.

Simon Modi MB BS, MRCP is Specialist Registrar in Cardiology at The Liverpool Heart and Chest Hospital, Liverpool, UK.

Acknowledgements

We would like to acknowledge help from several colleagues who generously contributed interesting cases for this book. These include Dr Archie Rao, Dr Mark Hall, Dr Derick Todd, Dr Nick Beeching, Dr Chris Bellamy, Dr David Roberts, Dr Scott Murray, Dr Christopher Wong, Dr Dhiraj Gupta, Dr Lindsay Morrison, Mr Abbas Rashid and Mr Aung Oo.

We would also like to express our appreciation to Ms Shelley Chow and the production staff at World Scientific Publishing for their help, advice and expertise in producing this book in a truly professional and timely manner.

This 58-year-old man was involved in a car-jacking incident and suffered minor trauma to his limbs with bruising and skin abrasions. A cardiologist was asked to provide a medico-legal report on his health as the patient had been found to have an irregular pulse by his general practitioner.

During the consultation, the patient admitted to having become progressively more breathless on exertion over the past 18 months and had noticed some ankle swelling in the past six months. On examination, he had an irregular pulse and a tachycardia of 120 bpm. The jugular venous pressure was elevated to the angle of the jaw and he had marked hepatomegaly and bilateral leg oedema extending to just below knee level. There was reduced air entry at both lung bases. The ECG and chest X-ray are shown below. There was no significant past medical history except that he had been stabbed in the chest at the age of 15 years.

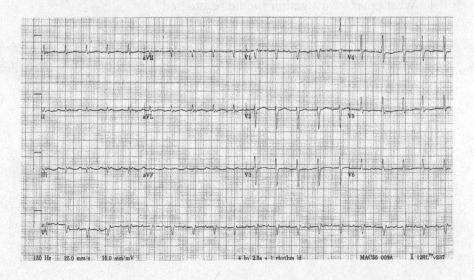

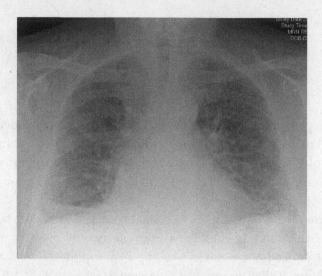

Questions:

1. What does the ECG show?
2. What does the chest X-ray show?
3. What initial treatment should be given?
4. What other investigation should be ordered?

Answers:

1. Cardiomegaly, pulmonary venous congestion, bilateral pleural effusions (right > left).
2. Atrial flutter with 2:1 block.
3. In-hospital bed rest, diuretics (intravenous or oral) and a rate controlling agent such as digoxin. Anticoagulant therapy should be commenced.
4. Echocardiography — to assess right and left ventricular function/ size, valve function, atrial size, presence/absence of septal defects or pericardial disease.

The echocardiogram was unremarkable and did not show any evidence of valvular disease or septal defects.

Question:

5. What further imaging test might be helpful?

Answer:

5. CT scan of the thorax.

The CT scan is shown here.

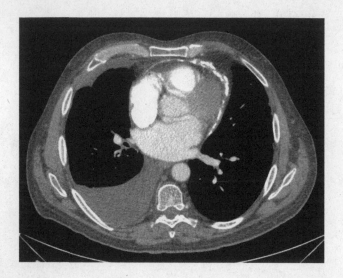

Q Questions:

6. What does the CT scan show?
7. What is the diagnosis?
8. What other investigation should be organised and what five characteristic features would confirm the diagnosis?
9. What treatment is appropriate?

Answers:

6. Dense pericardial calcification and right-sided pleural effusion.
7. Calcific constrictive pericarditis.
8. Cardiac catheterisation of the right and left heart (after stopping anticoagulants).

   (i)   Elevated right and left atrial pressures, elevated right and left ventricular end-diastolic pressures.
   (ii) Equalisation of RV and LV diastolic pressures; equalisation of RA and LA pressures.
   (iii) Rapid X and Y descent in RA and LA pressure trace.
   (iv) Typical "dip and plateau" waveform in RV and LV pressure recording.
   (v)   Increase in RA/LA/RVedp/LVedp with inspiration.

9. Pericardiectomy.

This 40-year-old man presented with left praecordial chest pain which was not regularly related to exertion. There were no abnormalities on physical examination and his resting ECG was normal. An exercise stress test produced −1.3 mm of upsloping ST-segment depression in V5 and V6 at a heart rate of 156 bpm in the third stage of a Bruce protocol. Diagnostic cardiac catheterisation was performed. Simultaneous injections into the right and left coronary artery (left lateral view) are shown below.

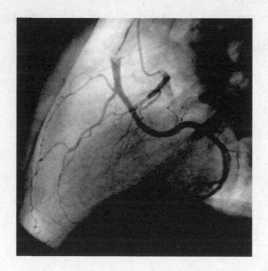

Questions:

1. What is the diagnosis?
2. What conclusions can be drawn from the investigation?

Answers:

1. Anomalous left circumflex coronary artery, originating from an ectopic, non-dominant right coronary artery.
2. The symptoms are not due to coronary artery disease. The exercise test should be regarded as a negative test.

A 60-year-old man required permanent pacemaker implantation.

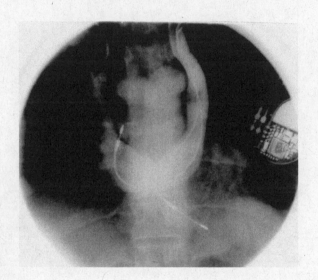

Q Questions:

1. What investigation has been performed here?
2. What abnormality is shown?
3. What specific precautions should be taken during the implantation procedure?

Answers:

1. Simultaneous contrast venography from catheters inserted into the right and left arms.
2. Right- and left-sided superior vena cava are present, only discovered during implantation of the first lead which took an abnormal course on fluoroscopy.
3. The pacemaker electrodes should be active fixation leads (particularly the atrial lead) in order to reduce the likelihood of lead displacement post-procedure.

A 74-year-old man presented with dyspnoea and fever of 38.8°C. The chest X-ray and CT scan are shown below.

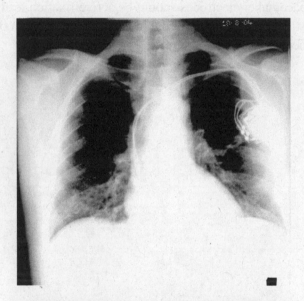

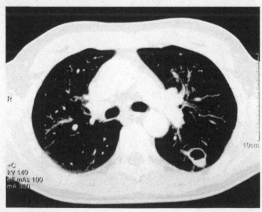

Questions:

1. What do the chest X-ray and the CT scan show?
2. What is the diagnosis and the likely cause?
3. What two investigations would you perform to confirm the diagnosis?
4. What is the treatment?

Answers:

1. The chest X-ray shows a permanent pacemaker with atrial and ventricular leads and a ring-shaped opacity in the left mid-zone.

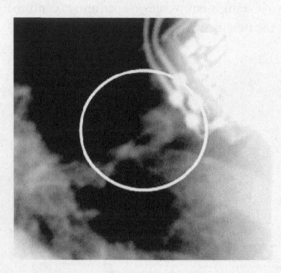

   The CT scan confirms that this is a cavity with a fluid level.
2. The diagnosis is pulmonary abscess, and the likely cause is infection of the pacing lead and/or the tricuspid valve resulting in septic pulmonary emboli. *Staphylococcus aureus* is the most likely organism in this patient whose pacemaker implantation took place seven weeks earlier.
3. (i) Blood cultures to identify the causative organism.
   (ii) Transoesophageal echocardiography is the best investigation to image the pacing leads and the tricuspid valve to look for infective vegetations.
4. Treatment consists of intravenous antibiotics and removal of the pacing system, especially if there is evidence of associated infection.

This 69-year-old male smoker complained of moderate effort breathlessness over the last year or so. He had no chest pain. Physical examination was unremarkable except that breath sounds were slightly reduced bilaterally. ECG showed sinus rhythm and no specific abnormalities. The chest X-ray (shown below) was thought to be abnormal and an echocardiogram and MRI scan were ordered.

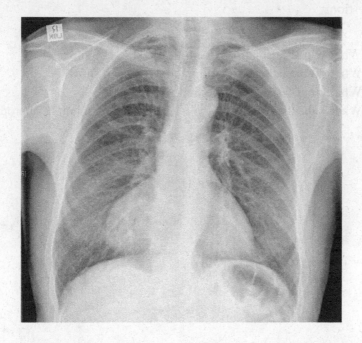

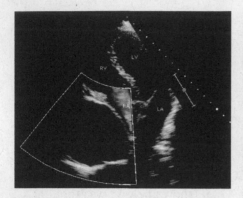 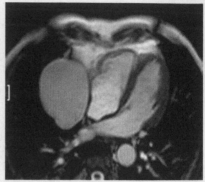

Q Questions:

1. What two abnormalities does the chest X-ray show?
2. What do the echocardiogram and MRI scan show?
3. What other tests should be done?
4. What is the likely diagnosis and what treatment might be appropriate?

Answers:

1. Hyperinflated lung fields and an abnormal enlargement of the right heart border.
2. The 2D echocardiogram shows a large fluid-filled mass within the pericardial space compressing the right atrium, and to a lesser degree, the right ventricle. Note the colour flow signal of blood across the tricuspid valve. The MRI scan shows the same cystic mass exhibiting mild compression of the right atrium.
3. Pulmonary function tests (PFTs).
4. The mass is a benign pericardial cyst. But the chest X-ray and subsequently the PFTs confirm obstructive airways disease. The cyst should be left alone and the obstructive airways disease may be treated with inhaled steroids and bronchodilators.

This 76-year-old man had a dual chamber permanent pacemaker implanted for complete heart block. A routine PA and lateral chest X-ray after the procedure is shown below along with his post-operative ECG.

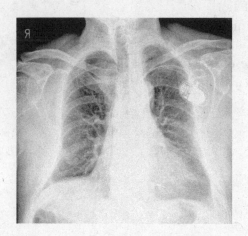
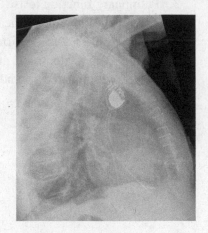

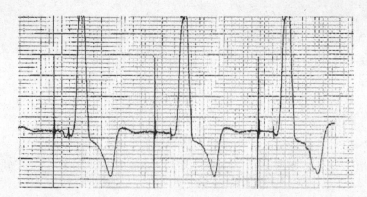

Questions:

1. What do the chest X-rays show?
2. What does the ECG show?
3. What should be done?

Answers:

1. Atrial lead displacement. This is best seen in the lateral X-ray.
2. Loss of atrial capture.
3. The atrial lead needs to be repositioned into the right atrial appendage.

Case **7**

A 65-year-old woman presented with acute onset chest pain, dyspnoea and sweating following the discovery of a burglary at her home. Her pulse was 150 bpm and BP 85/55 mmHg. A pan systolic murmur was audible over the praecordium. The ECG is shown below. A clinical diagnosis of post-infarct papillary muscle rupture/ dysfunction causing mitral regurgitation was made and cardiac catheterisation performed. Coronary arteriography was normal. The left ventricular angiogram showed only mild mitral regurgitation and its appearance in systole is shown below.

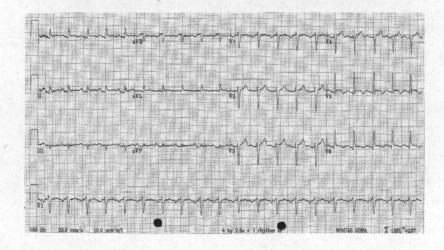

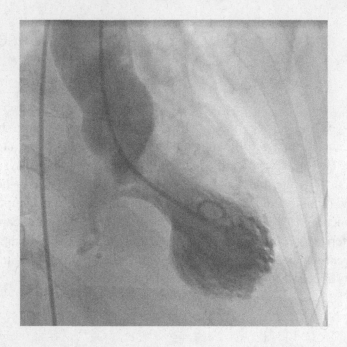

Questions:

1. What does the ECG show?
2. What does the left ventricular angiogram show?
3. What name has been attached to this condition?
4. What other investigation might be helpful?
5. What treatment should be given?

Answers:

1. Sinus tachycardia with non-specific ST- and T-wave abnormalities in the lateral chest leads but no evidence of acute myocardial infarction.
2. Apical ballooning of the left ventricle.
3. Takotsubo cardiomyopathy (named after the Japanese word for "octopus pot").
4. Echocardiography.
5. Intra-aortic balloon counterpulsation and inotropic support initially. Most cases are transient and recover with supportive measures only. Short- to medium-term therapy with angiotensin-converting enzyme (ACE) inhibitors and cardioselective β-blockers may be required when the condition stabilises.

This 67-year-old man was admitted to his local district general hospital with recurrent episodes of prolonged chest pain over a 24-hour period. He had hypercholesterolaemia and gout. His ECG showed ST-segment depression in leads V1–V4. The troponin T on admission was 0.77 μg/L and he was treated with aspirin, clopidogrel, bisoprolol, ramipril, atorvastatin, IV glyceryl trinitrate (GTN) and subcutaneous enoxaparin. At 12 hours the troponin T was >50 μg/L. He was referred for urgent cardiac catheterisation. The left coronary arteriogram is shown below (Left: right anterior oblique view; right: left lateral view).

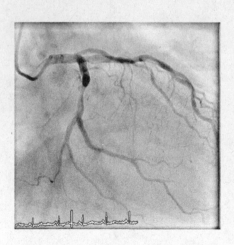 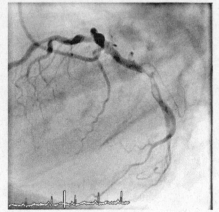

Questions:

1. What does the coronary angiogram show?
2. What additional medication should he be given?
3. What specific treatment is indicated?

Answers:

1. A severe, ulcerated stenosis in the proximal left circumflex (LCX) coronary artery with a large intracoronary thrombus attached to the stenosis and extending down the vessel.
2. The patient should be given IV or intracoronary unfractionated heparin and intracoronary/IV abciximab prior to percutaneous coronary intervention (PCI).
3. Thrombectomy using an aspiration catheter such as the Pronto™ device or a mechanical device such as the ThromCat™ should precede coronary stent implantation to the LCX lesion.

This 71-year-old man complained of breathlessness after walking 50 yards. His symptoms had been most noticeable for 18 months and were associated with chest tightness. He had had a myocardial infarction 12 years earlier and this was followed six months later by a stroke presenting as a right hemiparesis. Fortunately he recovered fully from the latter. His ECG is shown below and his chest X-ray showed cardiomegaly. Cardiac catheterisation was performed and systolic (left) and diastolic (right) frames from the left ventricular angiogram are shown below. Coronary arteriography showed severe right and left circumflex coronary artery disease and an occluded left anterior descending coronary artery.

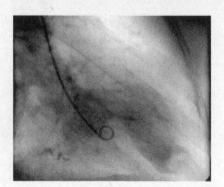 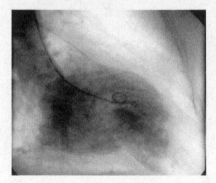

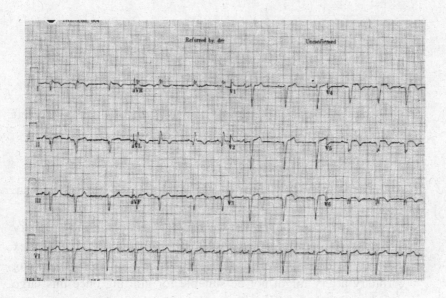

Q Questions:

1. What cardiac physical sign might be expected?
2. What two features are shown in the images?
3. What is the diagnosis?
4. What medical treatment is appropriate?
5. What other treatment should be considered?

Answers:

1. Paradoxical apical impulse.
2. Large anteroapical aneurysm and opacity at the apex of the left ventricle — best seen in the systolic (left) frame.
3. (i) Large left ventricular aneurysm.
   (ii) Left ventricular thrombus.
4. Anticoagulant therapy, diuretics, ACE inhibitor, β-blocker, aspirin, nitrate.
5. Surgical resection of the left ventricular aneurysm and coronary artery bypass grafting to the stenosed right and left circumflex coronary arteries. However, the occluded left anterior descending coronary artery might not be suitable for grafting once this large aneurysm has been resected.

This 45-year-old woman complained of breathlessness which had progressively worsened over the past nine months. A short, low-pitched diastolic murmur was noted by the cardiologist. The chest X-ray and pulmonary function tests were normal. The echocardiogram revealed the diagnosis.

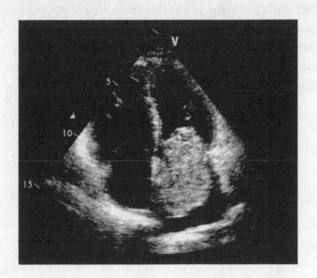

Q Questions:

1. What does the echocardiogram show?
2. What is the likely diagnosis?
3. What complications can occur?
4. What should be done?
5. What is the aetiology of the condition?

Answers:

1. A large, almost spherical, mass filling the left atrium and prolapsing across the mitral valve.
2. Left atrial myxoma.
3. Besides pulmonary congestion/oedema, the systemic complications can be serious and life-threatening. These include stroke, myocardial infarction and cardiac arrhythmias, bowel, splenic and renal infarction and peripheral limb ischaemia.
4. Surgical resection should be performed urgently since systemic embolisation of fragments of this often friable tumour can cause the disastrous complications outlined above.
5. Unknown at present. The development may be genetically determined as myxomas tend to occur in family members. They are more common in women than men.

Case 11

A 34-year-old lady presented to her general practitioner with a sore throat and temperature of 38.4°C. On examination, the tonsils were red and inflamed with yellow flecks of pus adherent to them. A systolic murmur was heard by the GP who referred her for a cardiology opinion. The cardiologist made the diagnosis on auscultation of the praecordium and confirmed it by echocardiography. The echocardiogram is shown below.

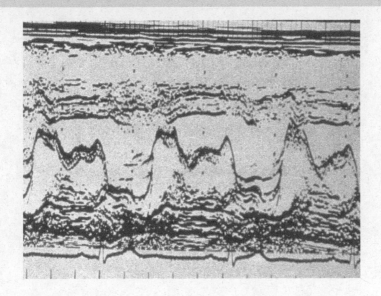

Questions:

1. What modality of echocardiography is this?
2. What is the diagnosis?
3. What auscultatory findings did the cardiologist record?

Answers:

1. An M-mode echocardiogram.
2. Mitral valve prolapse.
3. A mid-systolic click and late systolic murmur.

This young woman presented with malaise, loss of appetite, exertional dyspnoea, rigors and painful tender spots on the palmar and plantar aspects of the hands and feet respectively (shown below). She gave an eight-month history of progressively severe lower back pain. On admission, her temperature was 39.1°C and a pansystolic murmur was audible over the praecordium. The lumbar spine MRI is shown below.

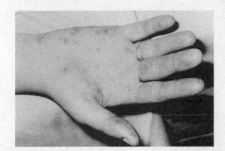
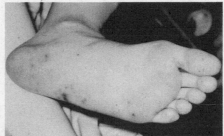

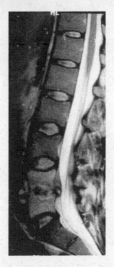

Questions:

1. What are the lesions on the hands and feet?
2. What does the MRI scan show?
3. What is the pansystolic murmur due to?
4. What is the likely diagnosis?
5. What are the two most important investigations necessary?
6. What is likely to be the cause for the pathology?

Answers:

1. Osler's nodes.
2. Discitis of L4/5. There is also spinal cord compression and vertebral osteomyelitis.
3. Mitral regurgitation.
4. Infective endocarditis.
5. Echocardiography and blood cultures.
6. *Staphylococcus aureus*.

This 57-year-old man developed severe dyspnoea 18 hours after an acute anterior myocardial infarction. The heart rate was 120 bpm and the BP 80/50 mmHg. A loud pansystolic murmur was audible over the praecordium. The chest X-ray and echocardiogram are shown below.

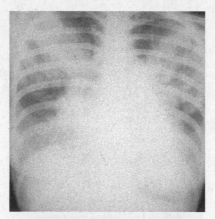

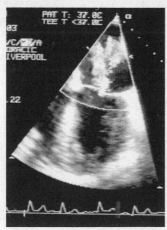

Questions:

1. What does the chest X-ray show?
2. What does the transoesophageal echocardiogram show?
3. What three specific treatments should be given immediately?
4. What other investigation should be performed?
5. What definitive treatment should be recommended?

Answers:

1. Acute pulmonary oedema.
2. Severe mitral regurgitation.
3. (i)   100% oxygen.
   (ii) Intravenous diuretics.
   (iii) Intra-aortic balloon counterpulsation.
4. Cardiac catheterisation and coronary arteriography.
5. Emergency mitral valve replacement and possibly concomitant coronary artery bypass surgery.

This 76-year-old West Indian man presented with a six-month history of increasing exertional dyspnoea and ankle swelling. He had no angina. He had been treated for pulmonary tuberculosis at the age of 19 years. On examination he looked well but the jugular venous pressure (JVP) was raised 6 cm. BP 150/85 mmHg, pulse 90 bpm, he had moderate ankle oedema and there was a soft mid-systolic murmur at the left sternal edge and apex. The ECG showed low voltage complexes and small R waves in V1–V4. The chest X-ray showed mild cardiomegaly and mild pulmonary venous congestion. The echocardiogram is shown below.

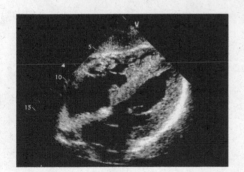 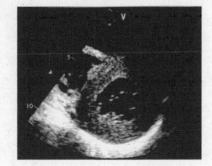

Questions:

1. What is the clinical diagnosis?
2. What does the echocardiogram show?
3. What is the pathophysiological explanation for the clinical findings? How can this be confirmed?
4. What is the likely aetiology?
5. What can be done to confirm the diagnosis?
6. What treatment is indicated?

Answers:

1. Congestive cardiac failure.
2. Globally increased thickness of right and left ventricular walls, increased atrial and ventricular septal thickness, "granular" or "sparkly" appearance to the myocardium.
3. Diastolic dysfunction causing restrictive defect. Doppler echocardiography should confirm impaired diastolic relaxation.
4. Primary cardiac amyloidosis.
5. Endomyocardial biopsy. Histology will show interstitial deposits of homogenous material which stains with Congo red and appears bright green under polarised light.
6. Symptomatic treatment with diuretics.

This is a chest X-ray of a 50-year-old woman who had presented to a cardiologist with odd intermittent "fainting attacks". Physical examination was normal as was the ECG.

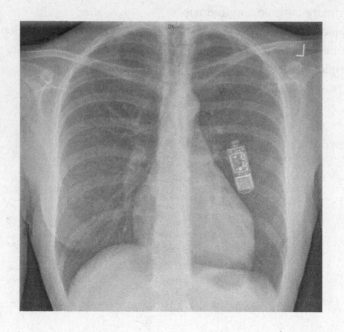

Q Questions:

1. What four cardiac investigations should be considered?
2. What does the chest X-ray show?
3. What test should be done before leaving hospital?

Answers:

1. (i)   Echocardiogram.
   (ii) Ambulatory ECG monitoring depending on the frequency of the attacks.
   (iii) If the latter fails to identify an arrhythmia, then an external loop recorder should be worn for two to three weeks. An event recorder might also be useful if prodromal symptoms are noticed.
   (iv) If these also fail to detect an arrhythmia, but the latter is seriously suspected, then an implantable ECG loop recorder should be inserted.
2. An implantable loop recorder (in this case a Reveal® device) has been subcutaneously implanted in the left parasternal region.
3. Care should be taken to position the device at an angle which provides an excellent ECG signal and this should be checked before leaving the operating theatre. The device can be programmed to automatically record prespecified dysrhythmias and/or patient-activated events using a small hand-held "activator". The stored arrhythmias can be subsequently identified by interrogating the device.

Case **16**

A 69-year-old man reported loss of consciousness whilst out walking. It occurred just as a fighter jet flew overhead at high speed. Physical examination was normal as was the 12-lead ECG.

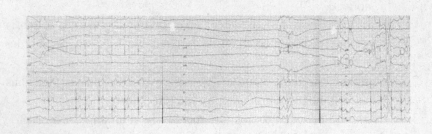

Questions:

1. What test has been performed here?
2. What does it show?
3. What is the diagnosis?
4. What treatment should be offered?

Answers:

1. Carotid sinus massage.
2. Sinus arrest occurs after carotid sinus massage and produces near syncope.
3. Carotid sinus hypersensitivity. Presumably the same situation arose when he looked skyward at the jet overhead.
4. Either single chamber atrial or dual chamber pacemaker implantation should be offered if avoidance of provocative manoeuvres does not render him asymptomatic. Absence of documented AV block would predict safe and efficacious AAI pacing above DDD.

A 67-year-old man developed severe central chest pain when digging up a tree in his garden. The pain radiated up to his neck and down the left arm. He gave a history of hypertension, hypercholesterolaemia and previous smoking. BP was 170/110 mmHg; pulse 100 bpm; no cardiac murmurs were audible. The chest X-ray on admission, ECG (one month before presentation) and CT scan (six hours after admission) are shown below.

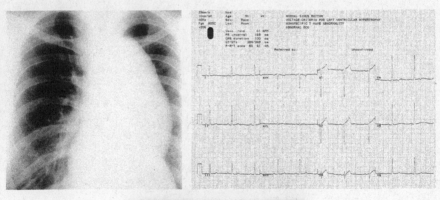

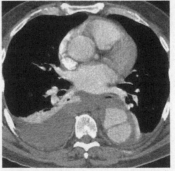

Q

Questions:

1. What do the three illustrations show?
2. What is the diagnosis?
3. What four other clinical features should be looked out for?
4. What treatment should be given immediately?
5. What three other investigations might be useful in such a patient?
6. What definitive treatment is indicated?

Answers:

1. The chest X-ray shows a widened mediastinum due to an enlarged thoracic aorta; the ECG shows left ventricular hypertrophy and the CT scan shows a dissection flap extending from the ascending to the descending thoracic aorta as well as an effusion in the right hemithorax — almost certainly a haemothorax.
2. Type I acute aortic dissection.
3. (i)   Unequal or missing pulses.
   (ii) Different BP in the two arms.
   (iii) Signs of aortic regurgitation.
   (iv) Symptoms or signs of ischaemia to bowel, kidneys or lower limbs.
4. Analgesia — IM/IV; β-blocker — IV and oral to reduce BP; IV nitrate or nitroprusside to reduce BP.
5. (i)   Echocardiography or CT scan. Both investigations showed that the dissection originated in the ascending aorta, just above the aortic valve.
   (ii) Aortography might be an option if CT/MRI were of poor quality or unavailable — not done in this case.
   (iii) Coronary arteriography might be necessary — after discussion with a cardiac surgeon.
6. Type I (intimal tear occurs in ascending aorta but extends into the descending aorta) and Type II (tear limited to ascending aorta) dissection — surgical repair.
   Type III (tear limited to descending aorta) — medical treatment initially; surgical treatment if evidence of bleeding, e.g. haemothorax, is found.

A 35-year-old female presented with a six-month history of short episodes of palpitations and sweating. A continuous praecordial murmur was audible. Aortography and transoesophageal echocardiography (TOE) confirmed the diagnosis. Images from both investigations are shown and the white arrow gives a clue to the diagnosis.

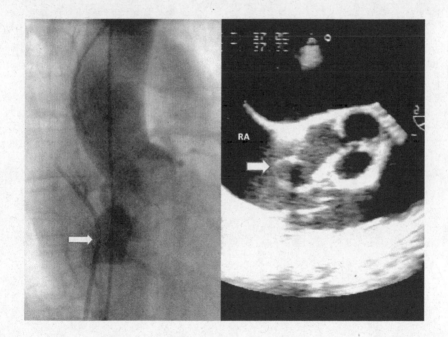

Questions:

1. What does the aortogram show?
2. What does the transoesophageal echocardiogram show?
3. What are the three possible aetiologies?
4. How else can we confirm the diagnosis?
5. What treatment should be offered?

Answers:

1. A ruptured sinus of Valsalva aneurysm.
2. Fistulous communication between the sinus of Valsalva and the right atrium.
3. (i)   Congenital.
   (ii) Infective endocarditis.
   (iii) Trauma.
4. CT scan; MRI scan.
5. Surgical repair.

A 26-year-old man was admitted with severe pain and swelling in his right arm at a site where he had been injecting IV heroin. He had been "shooting up" drugs since the age of 17 years. On examination, he was unwell, emaciated and pyrexial with a temperature of 38.9°C. He had a large painful swelling in the right antecubital fossa associated with marked oedema and cellulitis. Shortly after admission into hospital he had a rigor, his temperature rose to 39.9°C and he complained of sharp right-sided chest pain on coughing. Physical examination revealed a raised JVP, BP 110/60 mmHg, heart rate 128 bpm. Auscultation of the praecordium revealed a soft pansystolic murmur at the left sternal edge. There were crepitations audible over both right and left mid zones but generally good air entry on inspiration. A picture of his right arm and his chest X-ray are shown below.

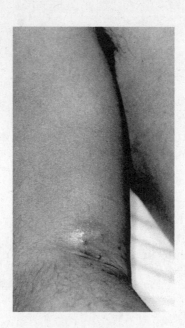

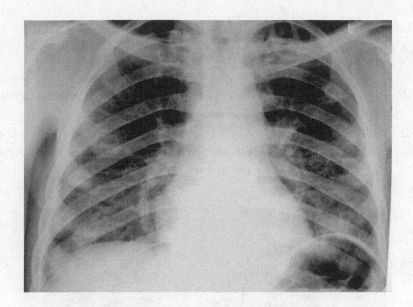

Questions:

1. What is the likely cause of the swelling in his right arm?
2. What does the chest X-ray show?
3. What five important tests should be carried out without delay?
4. What is the likely diagnosis?
5. What treatment is indicated?

Answers:

1. *Staphylococcus aureus* abscess in the right arm as a result of using dirty needles for IV drug abuse.
2. Multiple pulmonary abscesses. The typical appearance of a rounded opacity with both air and a fluid level is seen in the right mid zone (indicated by the arrow).

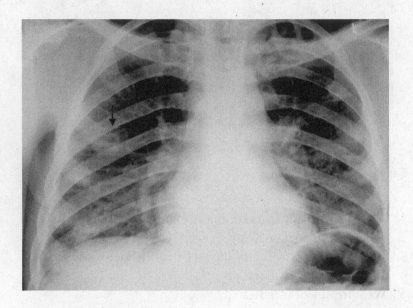

3. (i)   Full blood count, ESR, CRP.
   (ii) Blood cultures.
   (iii) Culture and sensitivity of pus from arm abscess.
   (iv) Echocardiography/transoesophageal echocardiography.
   (v)   CT scan of chest and abdomen.
4. Infective endocarditis of the tricuspid valve due to IV drug abuse, complicated by infected pulmonary emboli causing multiple lung abscesses. This is due to *Staphylococcus aureus* which was found in both the arm abscess and in the blood cultures.

5. Surgical drainage of the arm abscess; high dose IV flucloxacillin and IV fusidic acid initially, or IV vancomycin in penicillin-sensitive patients. Antibiotics may need to be changed depending on the results of microbiological culture and sensitivity testing. Continued observation of the patient with repeat blood tests, chest X-ray and echocardiograms is essential. If pulmonary abscesses continue to recur, the tricuspid valve vegetations fail to diminish or indeed enlarge despite antibiotics, then vegetectomy or tricuspid valve replacement may be necessary.

This 80-year-old lady had recurrent burning chest discomfort 15 years after undergoing coronary artery bypass surgery (CABG) surgery. Her symptoms were particularly troublesome when lying in bed. She remained symptomatic despite full antianginal treatment and thus cardiac catheterisation was performed to help decide whether percutaneous coronary intervention (PCI) or further surgical intervention might be helpful. The illustrations below show a right anterior oblique (left) and left lateral (right) fluoroscopic image just prior to the left ventricular angiogram, with the pigtail catheter *in situ*.

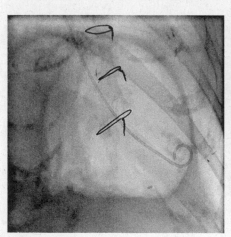 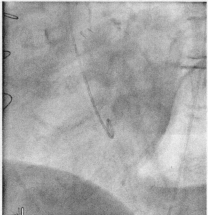

Questions:

1. What do the images show?
2. What is the diagnosis?
3. What treatment should be offered?

Answers:

1. A large globular radiolucent area overlying the cardiac silhouette.
2. Large hiatus hernia. The lucency can be seen to be behind the heart on the lateral view, distinguishing it from a large amount of air within the heart or pericardium.
3. A proton pump inhibitor and Gaviscon might help relieve symptoms of reflux. Surgical repair should probably be the last resort in this 80-year-old. The angiography showed that further coronary intervention was not necessary.

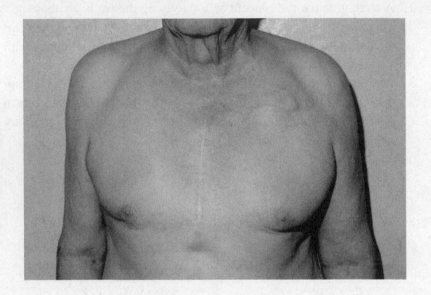

Questions:

1. What four features can be seen in the photo?
2. What is the diagnosis?
3. What is likely to be responsible for the pathology?
4. What treatment is necessary?

Answers:

1. (i) Mid-line sternotomy scar.
   (ii) Permanent pacemaker scar.
   (iii) Dilated veins over left pectoral region and engorged left external jugular vein.
   (iv) Swollen left arm.
2. Left subclavian vein thrombosis.
3. The two electrodes from the permanent pacemaker have resulted in thrombosis of the left subclavian vein at the insertion point.
4. Anticoagulation with warfarin in the first instance.

A 25-year-old woman complained of breathlessness, which was diagnosed as asthma by her general practitioner. She was referred to a chest physician for advice. The chest X-ray is shown below.

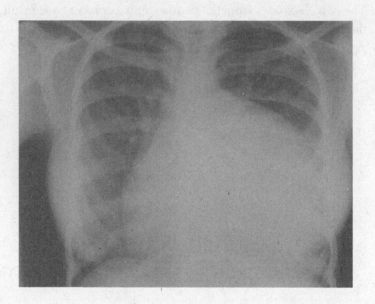

Questions:

1. What does the chest X-ray show?
2. What are the three possible causes?
3. What are the two most useful investigations?

Answers:

1. Massive cardiac silhouette.
2. (i) Large pericardial effusion.
   (ii) Thymoma.
   (iii) Dilated cardiac chambers, e.g. left atrium, right atrium, right ventricle and left ventricle.
3. Apart from physical examination:

   (i) Echocardiography.
   (ii) CT or MRI scan.

Case 23

This 39-year-old man had a sudden blackout at home, fell and fractured his clavicle. He complained of effort breathlessness, difficulty in walking and poor vision. His ECG is shown below (rhythm strip).

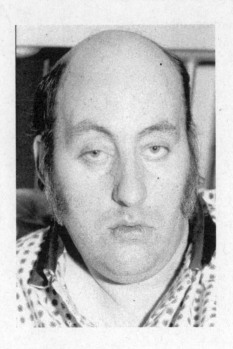

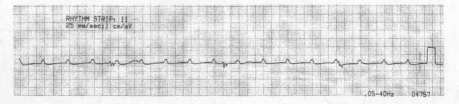

RHYTHM STRIP: II
25 mm/sec;1 cm/mV

.05-40Hz   04757

Q
Questions:

1. What is the diagnosis?
2. What three facial features typify the condition and are evident in the photo?
3. What does the ECG show?
4. What treatment is necessary in this case?

Answers:

1. Dystrophia myotonica.
2. (i)   Frontal balding.
   (ii) Bilateral ptosis.
   (iii) Long, haggard-looking expression.
3. Complete heart block.
4. Dual chamber permanent pacemaker implantation.

This 72-year-old man gave an eight-week history of anorexia, malaise, weight loss and low grade pyrexia but developed progressive dyspnoea over the past ten days prior to admission. He looked pale and his fingers are shown below. A short early diastolic murmur and a separate mid-diastolic murmur were audible over the praecordium.

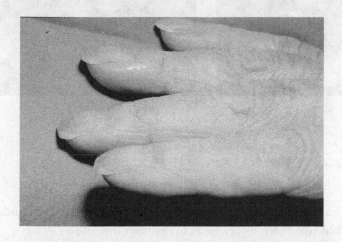

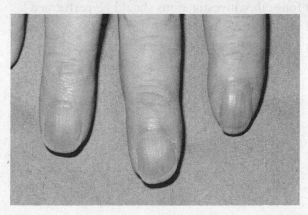

An echocardiogram was performed and two apical four-chamber views are shown below.

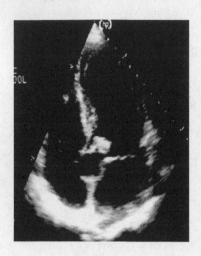 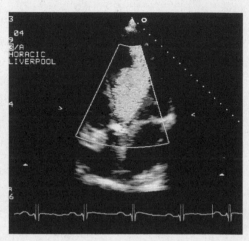

Q Questions:

1. What two physical signs are visible on examining the hands?
2. What two features do the echocardiograms show?
3. What four other investigations should be performed?
4. What medical treatment should be given?
5. What other treatment is necessary?

Answers:

1. Clubbing and splinter haemorrhages.
2. Large vegetation on the aortic valve and severe aortic regurgitation (colour flow).
3. (i)   Full blood count.
   (ii) CRP and ESR.
   (iii) Blood cultures.
   (iv) Coronary arteriography with a view to surgery.
4. High dose of IV antibiotics, e.g. 3G Benzylpenicillin IV qds and Gentamicin 80 mg tds IV until culture and sensitivity results are available.
5. Aortic valve replacement.

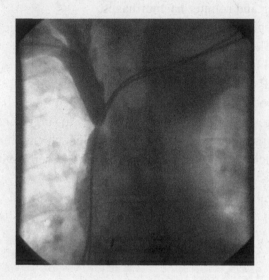

Q Questions:

1. What investigation has been performed here?
2. What does it show?
3. What is the cause?
4. What symptoms and physical signs might be expected?
5. What needs to be done?

Answers:

1. Venogram of the superior vena cava (SVC) via a catheter placed in the right arm.
2. The image shows a severe stenosis in the SVC.
3. Fibrosis due to adherence of two pacing electrodes to the wall of the SVC.
4. Headache, facial swelling, suffusion of the face, distended veins in the neck and upper chest wall, possible swelling of the arms.
5. Asymptomatic patients should simply be anticoagulated. In patients with clinical signs and symptoms, balloon dilatation of the stenosis should relieve the symptoms and signs of SVC obstruction. Stent implantation in the SVC might be effective if there is recurrent stenosis after balloon dilatation but may compromise the integrity of the pacing leads. Long-term anticoagulant therapy is indicated.

A 77-year-old man complained of breathlessness on minimal effort over the past five years. He had smoked 30 cigarettes per day since he was 23 years of age. He worked as a bookbinder for most of his working life. He was receiving no treatment at the moment. His general practitioner referred him for a cardiologist's opinion because of an apparent abnormally small heart on the chest X-ray. The chest X-ray and pulmonary function tests are shown below.

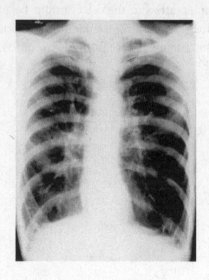

FVC: 2.1 L (pred 5.1 L)
FEV1: 1.0 L (pred 4.1 L)
PEFR: 4.1 L/sec (pred 9.2 L/sec)
FEV1/FVC: 47.6% (pred 80.1%)
TLC: 8.1 L (pred 7.2 L)
RV: 5.4 L (pred 2.6 L)
DLCO: 12.2 mL/min/mmHg (pred 30.4)

Q
Questions:

1. What three features does the chest X-ray show?
2. What do the pulmonary function tests show?
3. What is the diagnosis?
4. What treatment can be offered?

Answers:

1. Hyperinflated lung fields, low flat diaphragms and small cardiac silhouette.
2. Reduced FVC; reduced FEV1; reduced FEV1/FVC ratio; reduced peak expiratory flow rate (PEFR); increased total lung capacity (TLC); increased residual volume (RV); reduced transfer factor.
3. Emphysema.
4. Bronchodilator therapy, e.g. salbutamol, atrovent; domiciliary oxygen.

A 60-year-old man presented with angina of effort and exertional syncope. Physical examination revealed a small volume, anacrotic carotid pulse and an ejection systolic murmur at the left sternal edge. The left lateral chest X-ray taken after a "barium swallow" and the M-mode echocardiogram are shown below.

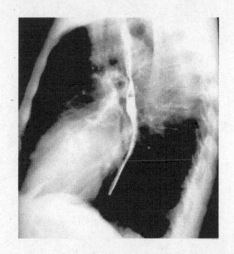

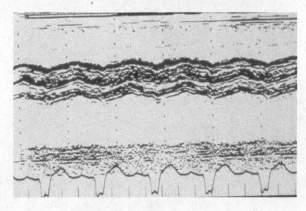

Questions:

1. What does the chest X-ray show?
2. What does the echocardiogram show?
3. What is the diagnosis?
4. What should be done next?
5. What definitive treatment is required?

Answers:

1. A ring of calcification is visible in the region of the aortic valve. Barium has been ingested to delineate the oesophagus.
2. Heavy calcification is present on the aortic valve obscuring the valve leaflets.
3. Calcific aortic stenosis.
4. Transthoracic echocardiography to assess the severity of the aortic stenosis and cardiac catheterisation to check the coronary anatomy. A left ventricle-aorta pullback gradient should only be performed if doubt exists over the severity of the stenosis.
5. Aortic valve replacement.

This 66-year-old former merchant seaman complained of dull, substernal pain. His symptoms occurred both at rest and on effort, especially at night. More recently, he had noticed a persistent cough and some hoarseness in his voice. He smoked 20 cigarettes per day. Physical examination revealed an ejection systolic murmur over the aortic area and an early diastolic murmur at the left sternal edge. The ECG showed sinus rhythm, left ventricular hypertrophy, ST-segment depression and T-wave inversion in leads V5–V6, leads I and AVL. The chest X-ray is shown below.

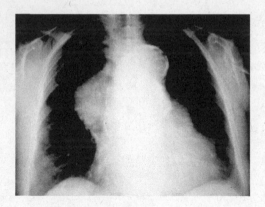

Q Questions:

1. What does the chest X-ray show?
2. What is the likely diagnosis?
3. What three tests are indicated?
4. What treatment should be offered?

Answers:

1. Cardiac enlargement; aneurysmal dilatation of the ascending aorta; thin, linear calcification of the ascending aorta extending down into the root.
2. Given his previous occupation, syphilitic aortitis and aortic regurgitation would be most likely.
3. (i)   Serology (TPHA, FTA-abs).
   (ii) Echocardiography.
   (iii) Cardiac catheterisation, including aortography and coronary arteriography.
4. Aortic root and valve replacement, possibly with concomitant coronary artery bypass surgery.

This 18-year-old man was found to be hypertensive (BP 185/105 mmHg) during a routine medical examination prior to army recruitment. He was not on any medical treatment. His chest X-ray is shown below.

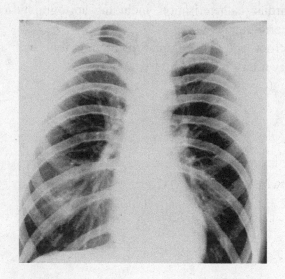

Q Questions:

1. What does the chest X-ray show?
2. What clinical features might be present?
3. What is the diagnosis?
4. What three investigations should be ordered?
5. What treatment is indicated?
6. What two conditions are associated with the diagnosis?

Answers:

1. Bilateral rib notching. Normal heart size.
2. (i)   Weak or impalpable femoral pulses.
   (ii) Radiofemoral delay.
   (iii) Palpable arterial pulsation over the scapulae.
   (iv) Systolic murmur over praecordium and over back.
3. Coarctation of the aorta.
4. (i)   Echocardiography.
   (ii) Cardiac catheterisation including aortography and an assessment of gradient across the coarctation.
   (iii) MRI with 3D reconstruction of the thoracic aorta.
5. Surgical resection with end-to-end anastomosis or tube graft interposition depending on anatomy. Balloon dilatation and stenting may be an alternative.
6. Bicuspid aortic valve and cerebral "berry" aneurysms.

This 56-year-old lady complained of breathlessness after doing her housework and shopping, walking more than 200 yards or climbing stairs. Her symptoms had developed over the last three years and especially over the past six months. As a girl, she suffered chorea and had a six-month period of bed rest in hospital. On examination, she looked well, pulse 100 bpm irregular, JVP normal, BP 140/80 mmHg. Auscultation revealed a loud first heart sound, an apical mid-systolic murmur and a mid-diastolic murmur. She had mild ankle oedema. Her ECG showed atrial fibrillation. The chest X-ray is shown below. An echocardiogram (recorded six months earlier) and cardiac catheterisation done during this admission are also shown. The relevant haemodynamic trace is also presented.

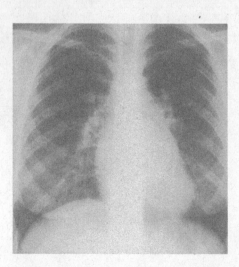
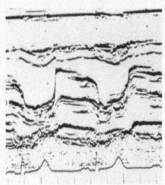

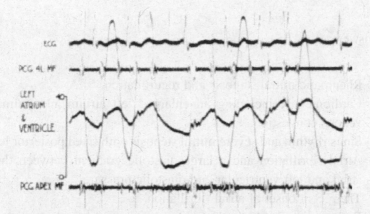

Q Questions:

1. What is the diagnosis?
2. What two features are present on the chest X-ray which are consistent with this diagnosis?
3. What does the echocardiogram show?
4. What does the catheter trace show?
5. What is the likely explanation for the recent deterioration?
6. What treatment should be considered?

Answers:

1. Rheumatic mitral stenosis and regurgitation.
2. Cardiomegaly including an enlarged left atrium and pulmonary venous congestion.
3. Sinus rhythm and severe mitral stenosis with fixed posterior leaflet.
4. Atrial fibrillation and a large diastolic gradient between the left atrial and left ventricular end-diastolic pressure.
5. The recent onset of atrial fibrillation.
6. Balloon mitral valvuloplasty (depending on the further echocardiographic features of the mitral valve and left atrium and the absence of significant mitral regurgitation) or mitral valve replacement. Direct current (DC) cardioversion to restore sinus rhythm following anticoagulation with warfarin.

This patient presented at the pacemaker follow-up clinic with no complaints.

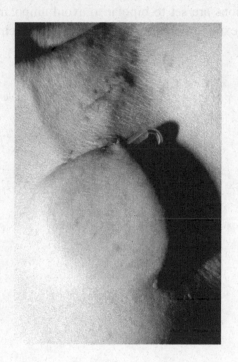

Questions:

1. What does the photograph show?
2. What needs to be done?

Answers:

1. Pacemaker lead erosion.
2. Removal of the entire pacing system and implantation of a new, subpectoral system on the contralateral side. Simply burying the lead will usually result in re-erosion or subsequent pocket infection. Until this can be performed it is imperative that lead configurations are set to bipolar to avoid unipolar loss of capture due to the extracorporeal location of part of the circuit.

A 44-year-old man had a five-week history of tight retrosternal chest pain on effort. His BP was 150/90 mmHg, heart rate 70 bpm, heart sounds were normal. His cholesterol was 6.8 mmol/L. The resting ECG was normal. An exercise stress test produced chest pain within two minutes of the Bruce protocol, hypotension and the ECG is shown below. Following sublingual glyceryl trinitrate, the ECG normalised (shown below). Urgent coronary angiography was performed and the salient feature is shown.

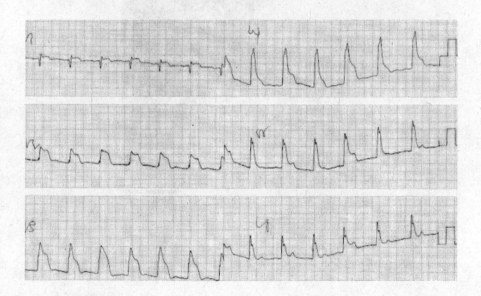

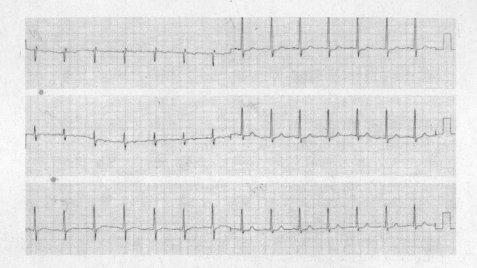

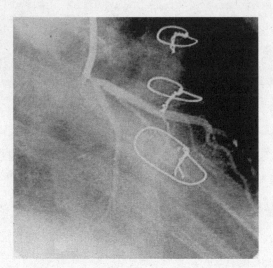

Questions:

1. What does the first ECG show?
2. What does it suggest?
3. What does the coronary angiogram show?
4. What treatment is indicated?

Answers:

1. Widespread acute anterior ST-segment elevation.
2. Extensive anterior myocardial ischaemia.
3. Severe left main stem stenosis.
4. Urgent coronary artery bypass surgery or percutaneous coronary intervention with drug-eluting stent implantation to the left main coronary artery.

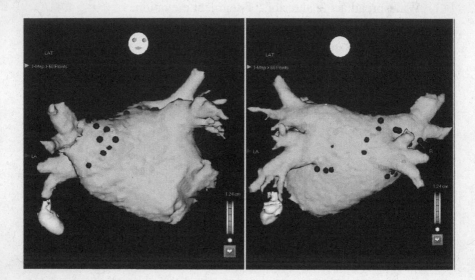

Q Questions:

1. What are these two images?
2. How have they been obtained?
3. What do the red dots signify?
4. What procedure has been performed?
5. How does the procedure work?
6. What are three potential complications of the procedure and their approximate frequency?

Answers:

1. These are CT images of the left atrium and pulmonary veins, as seen from the front and rear.
2. They have been obtained using the Carto XP EP Navigation System in combination with the CartoMerge Image Integration Software Module from Biosense Webster. This allows merging of pre-acquired 3D images of the chamber of interest (from CT or MRI scanner) with the electroanatomical data from the Carto XP EP system.
3. The red dots indicate where ablation lesions have been delivered using radiofrequency energy from the catheter's electrode.
4. Catheter ablation for atrial fibrillation, also known as pulmonary vein isolation.
5. Most cases of atrial fibrillation result due to rapidly firing electrical activity from one or more of the pulmonary veins. Current catheter ablation techniques involve electrically isolating these veins from the body of the left atrium so that these electrical impulses can no longer reach the atria and cause atrial fibrillation. This is achieved by creating burns using radiofrequency energy delivered by means of a catheter introduced via the peripheral venous system, right atrium and into the left atrium using an inter-atrial septal puncture (so-called trans-septal puncture) technique.
6. (i) Pulmonary vein stenosis following delivery of radiofrequency energy too far inside the pulmonary veins. This results in back pressure in the pulmonary venous system.
   (ii) Periprocedural stroke occurs in one in 200 cases.
   (iii) Cardiac tamponade occurs in one in 100 cases.

This 36-year-old man complained of having a syncopal episode during a game of squash. He had noticed increasing effort breathlessness over the past year or so and more recently of chest discomfort and mild dizziness during games of squash with his younger brother. Physical examination revealed a harsh ejection systolic murmur which was loudest at the left sternal edge and apex. The chest X-ray showed cardiomegaly and the ECG, phonocardiogram and echocardiogram (M-mode and 2D) are shown below.

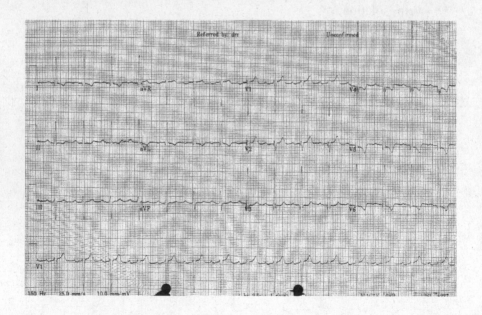

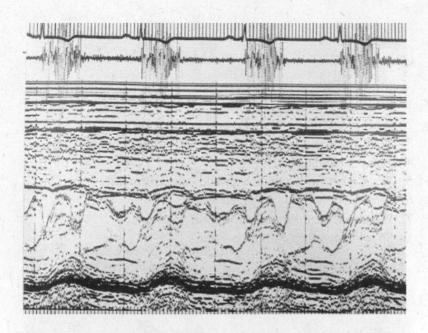

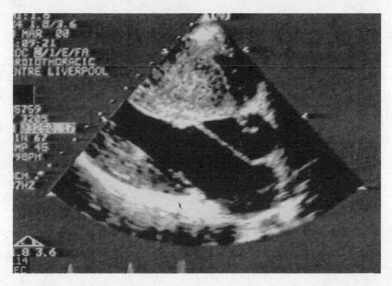

Questions:

1. What does the ECG show?
2. What two features does the echocardiogram show?
3. What other feature should be sought using echocardiography?
4. What is the diagnosis?
5. What other investigations should be performed?
6. What advice should be given?
7. What treatment should be offered?
8. Should any other advice be given?

Answers:

1. Sinus rhythm, left ventricular hypertrophy and left axis deviation.
2. (i) Severe asymmetric septal hypertrophy.
   (ii) Systolic anterior motion of the mitral valve.
3. Left ventricular outflow tract gradient should be sought.
4. Hypertrophic obstructive cardiomyopathy.
5. 24-hour ECG Holter monitoring; cardiac catheterisation and coronary arteriography; exercise testing to assess BP response.
6. Stop playing squash and other strenuous exertion.
7. He should be commenced on a β-blocker and considered for septal ablation/myomectomy and automatic implantable cardioverter defibrillator insertion.
8. His family members should be screened for hypertrophic cardiomyopathy.

A 32-year-old man presented with anorexia, weight loss, breathlessness over the last three days and tender red spots on his fingers and toes. He had a pyrexia of 39.1°C and intermittent rigors. He had a bounding pulse 100 bpm and the BP was 135/40 mmHg. A midsystolic and early diastolic murmur were audible at the left sternal edge. His ECG showed sinus tachycardia and the chest X-ray showed cardiomegaly and mild pulmonary oedema. Examination of the fundi revealed an unusual appearance and is shown below.

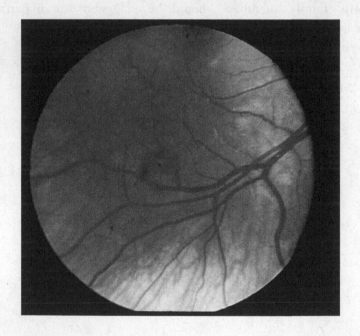

Q
Questions:

1. What does the picture show?
2. What is the likely diagnosis?
3. What five investigations would help make the diagnosis?
4. What two important questions should he be asked?
5. What is the cardiac diagnosis?
6. What immediate treatment is necessary?
7. What further treatment is likely to be required?
8. What ECG parameter should be monitored during his treatment?

Answers:

1. Roth spot.
2. Infective endocarditis
3. (i) Full blood count.
   (ii) CRP/ESR.
   (iii) Blood cultures.
   (iv) Transthoracic echocardiography.
   (v) Transoesophageal echocardiography.
4. (i) Is he an intravenous drug abuser?
   (ii) Has he had any dental or surgical procedures performed recently?
5. Severe aortic regurgitation.
6. IV antibiotics — 3G qds IV Flucloxacillin, 3G four-hourly IV Benzylpenicillin, IV Gentamicin 120 mg eight-hourly initially until blood cultures reported.
7. Aortic valve replacement.
8. PR interval due to the development of an aortic root abscess compressing or invading the atrioventricular node.

A 78-year-old man presented with increasing shortness of breath on exertion. He had neither cough nor chest pain, but had lost a significant amount of weight over the past six months. His appetite was reasonable and there were no other gastrointestinal symptoms. He had chronic obstructive airways disease. He gave a previous history of bladder cancer and underwent annual cystoscopy.

On examination, he was cachectic. His pulse was 70 bpm and BP 120/70 mmHg. His jugular venous pressure was elevated with a prominent V wave. A right ventricular heave was detected. Auscultation revealed a pansystolic murmur audible all over the praecordium. Respiratory examination revealed good air entry with expiratory wheeze and no crepitations. He had moderate pitting ankle oedema.

An ECG showed atrial fibrillation and right bundle branch block. The echocardiogram is shown below.

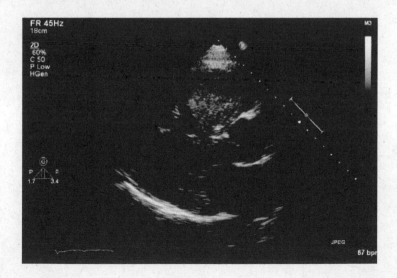

Questions:

1. What does the echocardiogram show?
2. What is the differential diagnosis?
3. What investigations should be considered next?
4. What is the definitive treatment?

Answers:

1. A large globular mass in the right ventricle.
2. Tumour, e.g. myxoma, lipoma, teratoma, metastasis, sarcoma; large thrombus.
3. Transoesophageal echocardiography, CT or MRI for characterisation of the mass and its anatomy; cardiac catheterisation as a prelude to cardiac surgery, e.g. for coronary arteriography.
4. Surgical excision.

A 56-year-old male shop worker gave a year long history of increasing shortness of breath and central chest pain on exertion, such as climbing stairs. He had previously been investigated for chronic diarrhoea and abdominal pains with no abnormalities detected. He had a long history of bouts of pain in both hands and feet. He was a non-smoker and there was no family history of ischaemic heart disease. He had a younger brother with renal failure requiring dialysis and his father died aged 44 years of a cerebrovascular accident. His son complained of post-prandial abdominal pain and bloating.

On examination, his blood pressure was 118/78 mmHg. Cardiovascular examination revealed a prominent apex beat and a grade 2/6 ejection systolic murmur loudest at the left sternal edge. The character of the pulse was normal. Abdominal examination revealed small raised red skin lesions and mild tenderness in the epigastrium. Urine dipstick showed significant proteinuria.

Initial investigations included an ECG (shown). Respiratory function tests were normal. Echocardiogram revealed left ventricular hypertrophy with normal systolic function and no valvular abnormalities. This was confirmed at cardiac catheterisation when normal coronary anatomy was also demonstrated.

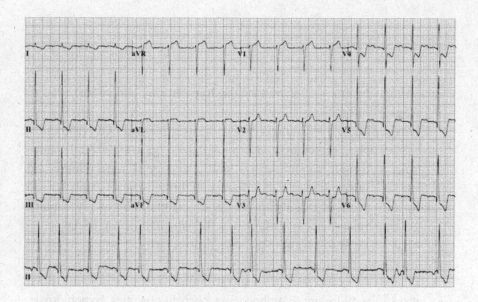

Questions:

1. What does the ECG show?
2. What are the skin lesions?
3. What is the most probable diagnosis?
4. How would you confirm this diagnosis?
5. What is the mode of inheritance?
6. What other complications may occur?
7. What treatment should be considered?

Answers:

1. Voltage criteria for left ventricular hypertrophy and strain.
2. Angiokeratomas.
3. Fabry disease. The combination of unexplained left ventricular hypertrophy, proteinuria and unexplained gastrointestinal symptoms in a male patient with a family history of renal failure and stroke is suggestive of Fabry disease. Fabry disease is characterised by deficiency of α-galactosidase and accumulation of glycosphingolipids in cardiac, vascular, renal, hepatic and neural tissue.
4. Measurement of serum α-galactosidase activity.
5. X-linked recessive.
6. Besides the acroparaesthesia and angiokeratomas, proteinuria, renal insufficiency/failure, lymphoedema, corneal opacities, hypohidrosis, stroke, myocardial infarction and heart failure may occur.
7. Enzyme replacement therapy using two-weekly IV infusion of either Agalsidase beta (Fabrazyme®) or Agalsidase alfa (Replagal®).

This 20-year-old man had undergone replacement of his automatic implantable cardioverter defibrillator four weeks earlier. He had developed redness, tenderness and swelling around the device and a temperature of 38.5°C. His general practitioner gave him amoxicillin 500 mg qds for five days and then because of continued discomfort around the wound, he referred the patient to the cardiologist.

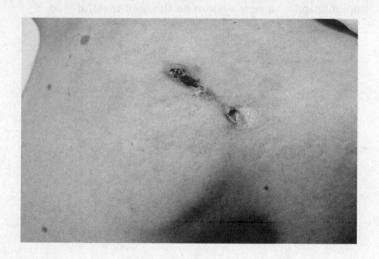

Questions:

1. What is the diagnosis?
2. What is the likely cause?
3. What three tests should be done?
4. What should be done next?
5. What additional procedure is necessary?

Answers:

1. Device-pocket infection.
2. *Staphylococcus aureus* is the most likely organism to infect so soon after the implantation procedure.
3. (i)   Full blood count.
   (ii) Blood cultures.
   (iii) Swab from the wound, if there is any discharge.
4. High dose IV flucloxacillin should be given for a minimum of two weeks.
5. Removal of the infected device and electrodes in their entirety and implantation of a new system on the contralateral side.

This 69-year-old man "blacked out" and fell into a pond in his garden. He regained consciousness soon after becoming submerged and called for help. Upon arrival at the hospital, he was fully conscious and symptom-free. His blood pressure was 125/75 mmHg and his pulse was irregular. An ECG confirmed atrial fibrillation with a rate of 78 bpm. There were no other abnormalities on physical examination, the chest X-ray showed slight cardiomegaly. He was taking bendrofluazide 2.5 mg daily for mild hypertension, digoxin 0.125 mg daily and warfarin. Investigations were organised and findings from the 24-hour ambulatory ECG are shown below. He was admitted to the hospital.

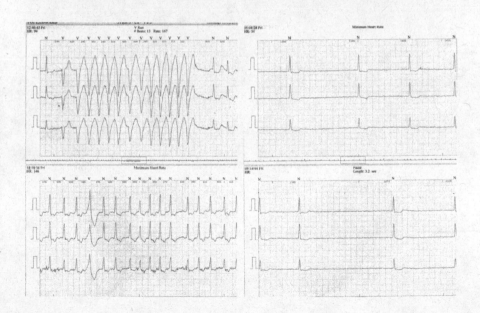

Questions:

1. What do the ECGs show?
2. What three investigations should be ordered on admission?
3. Based on the results of the initial investigations, what two other investigations should be considered?
4. What is the diagnosis?
5. What treatment should be offered?

Answers:

1. Non-sustained broad complex tachycardia (likely ventricular tachycardia or aberrantly-conducted atrial fibrillation) with underlying atrial fibrillation (left-upper panel); atrial fibrillation with fast ventricular rate (left-bottom panel); atrial fibrillation with slow ventricular response (right hand panels).
2. Serum electrolyte (potassium/magnesium) levels; digoxin level; echocardiogram.
3. Ventricular tachycardia (VT) stimulation study and coronary arteriography.
4. Tachy-brady syndrome is suggested by the presence of both slow and rapid ventricular rates in AF. However, the cause of the VT is unexplained.
5. Treatment hinges around the explanation of the broad complex tachycardia which looks suspiciously like VT. Assuming either a reversible cause for VT (e.g. digoxin toxicity, pause-dependent VT) or a "normal heart" VT, then one option would be pacemaker implantation. This option relies heavily on the assumption that the presenting syncope was unrelated to VT and more related to brady-cardia. If doubt or structural cardiac disease exists then AICD implantation might be more appropriate.

This 75-year-old man complained of effort breathlessness 15 years after coronary artery bypass surgery. He had impaired left ventricular function.

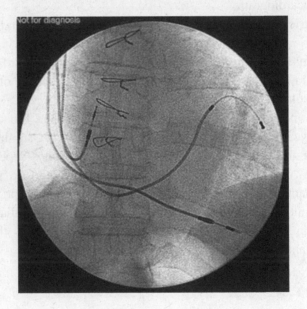

Q Questions:

1. What does the image show?
2. What procedure has been performed?
3. What four criteria should be evident before offering this treatment?
4. What additional criteria may be used to select patients?

Answers:

1. The image shows an actively-fixed pacing electrode in the right atrial appendage, a similar electrode in the right ventricular apex and a third electrode in the coronary sinus and passively fixed in a branch coronary vein; a previous sternotomy.
2. Cardiac resynchronisation therapy (CRT-P). The device is not shown.
3. (i) Symptomatic heart failure — New York Heart Association ≥ Class II.
   (ii) LVEF ≤ 35%.
   (iii) Broad QRS complex (> 150 ms — although some authorities are increasingly using 120 ms as a cut-off point).
   (iv) Optimal medical treatment.
4. Echocardiographic evidence of dyssynchrony in patients with QRS duration less than 150 ms.

This 69-year-old lady had an 18-month history of angina and progressive dyspnoea over the past two years. Her angina had deteriorated recently. She was taking atenolol for hypertension.

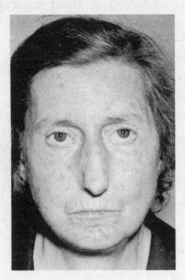 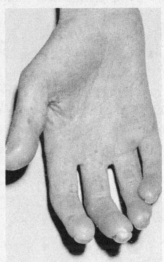

Questions:

1. What three features are shown by her face?
2. What does the hand show?
3. What is the diagnosis?
4. What is the likely cause of her dyspnoea?
5. What four investigations should be arranged?
6. What treatment could be offered?

Answers:

1. Fixed facial expression, telangiectasia, and small, puckered mouth.
2. Fixed flexion deformity, sclerodactyly (acrosclerosis), digital ulcer/ calcinosis at tip of the middle finger, telangiectasia on skin of palm and fingers.
3. Systemic sclerosis or scleroderma.
4. Pulmonary fibrosis (Thiebierge–Weissenbach syndrome).
5. Chest X-ray, pulmonary function tests, CT scan of thorax, and coronary arteriography.
6. The atenolol should be stopped and high-dose diltiazem should be used instead. This might help improve her symptoms of Raynaud's phenomenon. Steroids or other immunosuppressive agent may be required if pulmonary fibrosis is confirmed. Severe ostial lesions in the right and left main coronary arteries were found on further investigation and coronary artery bypass surgery was performed.

This 17-year-old male attended the general practitioner because of symptoms of breathlessness when cycling. His fellow cyclists commented that he looked "blue in the face" when on their normal 30 mile training run which involved hill cycling. His parents had told him that a heart murmur was diagnosed at birth but it was thought not to be of any significance and further investigations or medical examinations never took place. Physical examination revealed a harsh ejection systolic murmur — loudest at the upper left sternal border, fixed splitting of the second heart sound, and reduced intensity of the pulmonary component of the second heart sound. A fourth heart sound was audible at the lower left sternal border. The chest X-ray and ECG are shown below. Cardiac catheterisation was performed and the relevant information is also illustrated below.

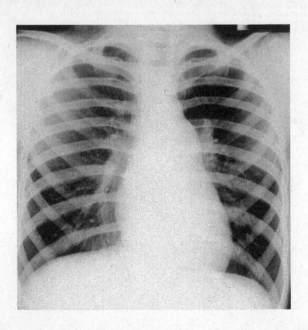

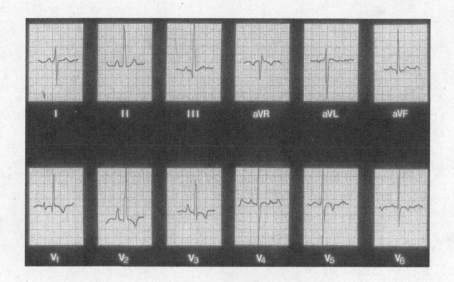

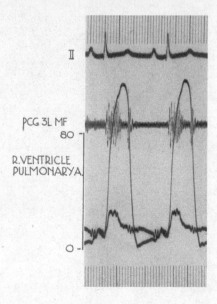

Q Questions:

1. What three other physical signs might be expected?
2. What does the chest X-ray show?
3. What three features does the ECG show?
4. What two other investigations might be helpful?
5. What does the catheter trace show?
6. What is the diagnosis?
7. What treatment should be recommended?

Answers:

1. Raised jugular venous pressure with a prominent "a" wave; right ventricular heave or parasternal lift due to right ventricular hypertrophy; systolic thrill over the second left intercostal space may also be palpable.
2. Slight cardiomegaly due to right ventricular enlargement, prominent pulmonary conus.
3. Tall peaked P waves due to right atrial hypertrophy; prominent R waves in V1 and right axis deviation due to right ventricular hypertrophy.
4. Echocardiography and cardiac catheterisation.
5. A systolic gradient of almost 100 mmHg across the pulmonary valve.
6. Severe pulmonary stenosis.
7. Balloon valvuloplasty of the pulmonary valve should be considered, although a homograft pulmonary valve replacement might be necessary.

This 57-year-old man with dyspnoea was found to have severe hypertension and sinus tachycardia and the skin lesions shown below.

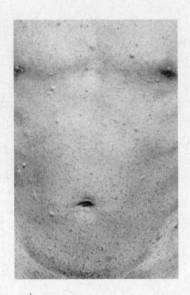

Q Questions:

1. What does the picture show?
2. What condition does he have?
3. On which chromosome has a mutation occurred?
4. What associated condition should be ruled out?
5. What tests should be requested?
6. Name four other cardiovascular pathologies that have been associated with his condition.

Answers:

1. Cutaneous neurofibromas.
2. Von Recklinghausen's disease or neurofibromatosis.
3. Chromosome 17.
4. Phaeochromocytoma.
5. 24-hour urinary catecholamine excretion and MRI of adrenal glands.
6. (i)   Cardiac rhabdomyoma.
   (ii) Primary pulmonary hypertension.
   (iii) Congestive cardiac failure.
   (iv) Arrhythmias.

A 36-year-old woman complained of palpitations and was found to have a narrow complex tachycardia of 220 bpm with no clearly discernable P waves.

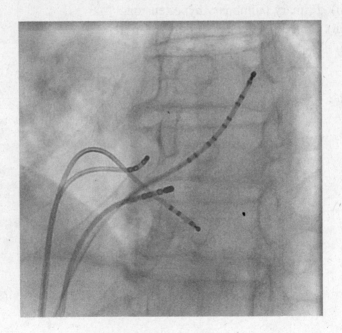

Q Questions:

1. What procedure is being performed?
2. What does the picture show?
3. What three arrhythmia types will this procedure help distinguish?
4. What are the five most common complications of this procedure?

A̶nswers:

1. An electrophysiological study +/– radiofrequency ablation.
2. Four electrodes positioned within the heart. Quadripolar catheters are placed in the right ventricular apex and adjacent to the bundle of His (upper tricuspid annulus) and a multipolar electrode is placed in the coronary sinus. The thicker tipped quadripolar ablation catheter appears to be positioned at the tricuspid annulus in the region of a "slow pathway".
3. (i) Atrial-driven arrhythmias such as atrial fibrillation, atrial flutter and atrial tachycardias.

   (ii) AV nodal re-entrant arrhythmias using dual AV nodal physiology (slow–fast AV nodal pathways).

   (iii) AV re-entrant arrhythmias using accessory pathways (e.g. overt (WPW syndrome), concealed or latent accessory pathways).
4. (i) Cardiac tamponade.

   (ii) AV node damage necessitating pacemaker implant.

   (iii) Pneumothorax (if subclavian or jugular access is used).

   (iv) Stroke (if left atrial access is obtained).

   (v) Vascular damage.

   Complications occur in approximately 1% of cases.

This 35-year-old man had a syncopal attack whilst running on the treadmill at the gym. His brother had died suddenly at the age of 28 years. An ECG taken in Accident and Emergency Department showed ventricular tachycardia with a rate of 230 bpm and a left bundle branch block (LBBB) morphology. The ECG below was recorded following DC cardioversion.

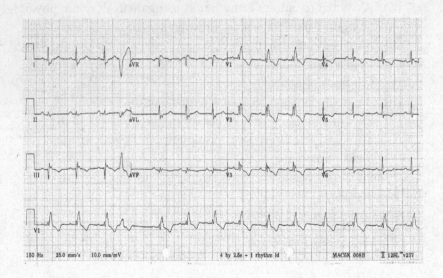

Q Questions:

1. Identify three major ECG abnormalities.
2. What investigation should he undergo next?
3. What is the likely diagnosis?
4. What treatment do you recommend?

Answers:

1. There is QRS widening in leads V_1–V_4 with a secondary R wave, akin to a right bundle branch block pattern. However, the QRS complexes in V_5 and V_6 appear narrow. Less extreme forms of this phenomenon are termed epsilon waves and represent RV late potentials. There is T wave inversion in leads V_1–V_4 and abnormal repolarisation in V_5–V_6. These features suggest a right ventricular pathology. The fourth beat of the recording is a ventricular ectopic. The morphology in lead V_1 (rhythm strip) in fact suggests it has a left ventricular or septal origin as it appears to have a right bundle branch block (RBBB) morphology. Its significance is debatable.

2. Echocardiography and cardiac MRI to look for right ventricular (RV) dilatation, RV dysfunction, fatty infiltration and microaneurysms.

3. Arrhythmogenic right ventricular cardiomyopathy (ARVC). ARVC is an inherited cardiomyopathy characterised by progressive fibro-fatty infiltration of the right ventricle. It is being increasingly identified as a cause of sudden cardiac death (SCD) in the young. Its clinical manifestations include ventricular arrhythmias (ectopy, VT and VF) and progressive right heart failure. Arrhythmias are often induced by exertion. It is inherited in an autosomal dominant fashion.

4. Automated implantable cardioverter defibrillator (AICD) implant. Although there are no large randomised clinical trials, current guidelines suggest that AICD implant is indicated in those patients in whom ARVC is diagnosed and who present with VF or sustained VT. AICD implant may also be indicated if there are high risk features (unexplained syncope, extensive right ventricular disease, LV involvement, family member with SCD). β-blockers are often used in an attempt to reduce the frequency of arrhythmia episodes, as is amiodarone, but there has been no systematic study to show benefit. ACE inhibitors are also used empirically in an attempt to slow the progression of the disease.

A 56-year-old man with previous history of myocardial infarction presented with increasing breathlessness. Examination revealed a raised JVP, pedal oedema and bilateral basal crackles in the lungs. His initial ECG is shown below. A subsequent echocardiogram confirmed severe impairment of LV systolic function with mild mitral regurgitation. He was commenced on medication for heart failure.

Despite this, he remained very symptomatic and continued to have limited exercise capacity. Following optimisation of his medication, an intervention was performed for him that improved his heart failure symptoms. A subsequent ECG is shown.

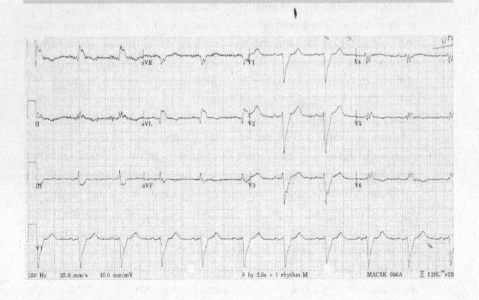

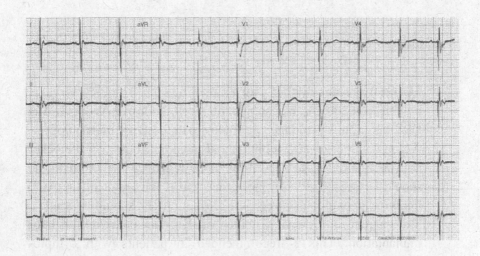

Questions:

1. What does the first ECG show?
2. What medication should be prescribed in heart failure?
3. What intervention was performed?
4. What does the second ECG show?

Answers:

1. ECG shows sinus rhythm with a rate of 60 bpm. The PR interval is prolonged at 200 ms, indicating borderline first-degree AV block. The QRS duration is prolonged at 166 ms with a LBBB morphology.

2. A loop diuretic, an ACE inhibitor and an optimal dose of a β-blocker such as bisoprolol or carvedilol. If he remained symptomatic he should be prescribed spironolactone and if intolerant of the ACE inhibitor an angiotensin receptor blocker (ARB) should be tried.

3. The patient underwent a biventricular pacemaker/defibrillator implantation. This is recommended in patients with symptomatic heart failure (despite optimal medication) and broad QRS complexes > 120 ms in an attempt to synchronise the right and left heart and optimise cardiac output.

4. The post-procedure ECG suggests atrial sensing and biventricular pacing. The pacing spike precedes each ventricular paced complex. Note that the AV delay is shorter than the intrinsic PR interval in order to facilitate pacing. The QRS complexes are narrow and the R–S ratio in Lead I is less than one, suggesting left ventricular capture.

A 45-year-old man attended pacing clinic for routine three-monthly interrogation of his defibrillator. His device was implanted two years previously and he had a number of antitachycardia pacing (ATP) therapies and shocks for ventricular tachycardia up until four months ago when he was started on amiodarone. He reported a recurrence of arrhythmias. Twenty episodes were recorded, an example of which is shown (top: atrial EGM; middle: A & V markers; lower: ventricular EGM). Subsequently a chest X-ray is done and is shown below. The technician states that the V lead impedance had risen from 1200 to > 2000 Ω.

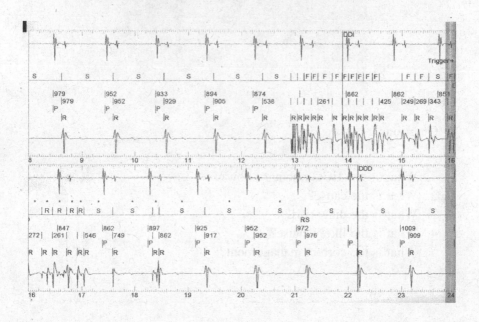

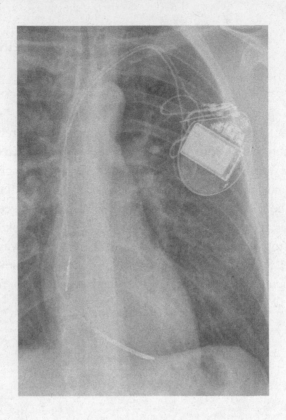

Q Questions:

1. What do the ECG tracings show?
2. What is the cause?
3. What is the diagnosis?
4. What is the likely cause?
5. What is the correct management?

Answers:

1. Oversensing on the V channel leading to R–R intervals within the VF detection zone. One can be confident about oversensing as the farfield V EGM seen on the atrial lead remains unchanged.
2. "Noise" on pacemaker leads often represents damage to either lead insulation or conductor. Header malconnections can also cause intermittent noise. Unipolar sensing can also pick up extraneous signals (e.g. myopotentials).
3. There is a clear conductor fracture in the ventricular pace/sense/shock lead seen just below the clavicle.
4. Given the position, compression and damage at the site of the pectoral securing-suture is likely.
5. Because of the history of recent/previous appropriate therapies for VT/VF the patient should be prioritised for lead replacement. Shock therapies should be deactivated due to the high probability of inappropriate shocks occurring. Inpatient cardiac monitoring would be recommended until this management is enacted.

A 60-year-old male underwent permanent pacemaker insertion for symptomatic complete heart block. A right atrial lead and right ventricular septal lead were positioned with good initial implant parameters. Post-operative chest X-ray shows the AP (below) and lateral position of the implant. The patient is discharged on the same day, but unfortunately returns with worsening symptoms and an episode of syncope. The chest X-ray is repeated but appears unchanged. Pacing parameters were unchanged but the technician commented that on the limb lead ECG taken at the time of the pacing check, AVL had an unusual "QS" paced appearance.

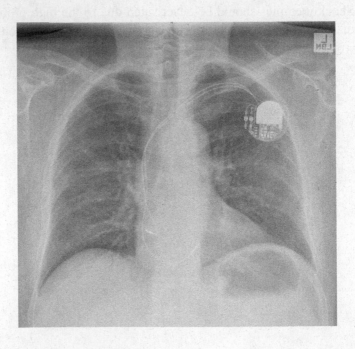

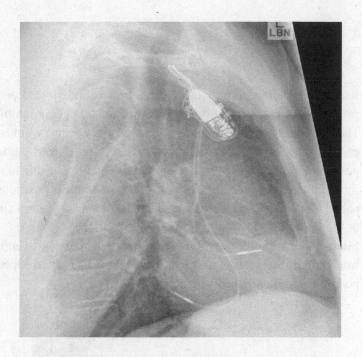

Q

Questions:

1. What is the initial differential diagnosis?
2. What is the likely problem?
3. What is the management?

Answers:

1. Intermittent failure to pace due to either micro/macro lead displacement, header malconnection or oversensing and pacing inhibition.
2. The original "septal" lead was placed in the coronary sinus. This can be seen in the lateral film with the "septal" lead's posterior positioning. Intermittent loss of capture is likely to be due to mobility within the coronary sinus in different anatomical positions. The paced QS in AVL is suggestive of a RBBB paced pattern (instead of the usual LBBB) due to initial LV activation.
3. Management should involve temporary increase in ventricular lead output, monitoring and lead reposition. Corrected septal lead position is shown below (arrow).

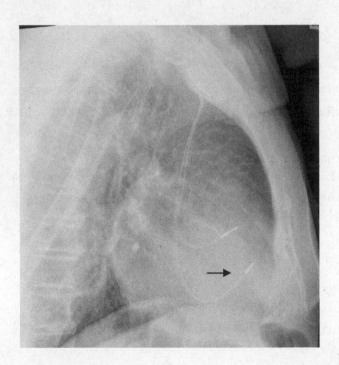

A 19-year-old student was referred for assessment of syncopal episodes. She was slim and active, participating in many university sports to first team level. Recently at the national university swimming semi-finals she was syncopal at the water's edge which alarmed her coach. Her team mates described pallor, rolling eyes and one suggested the presence of a very rapid weak pulse. The episode lasted between 30 and 60 seconds. She had had numerous other episodes, generally during competitions, although none quite this bad and was known to be a "fainter" during adolescence particularly around exam time. She was otherwise well, not on any medication and denied excessive alcohol intake or illicit drug use. A maternal aunt died aged 25 years as the sole occupant in a car crash and two cousins had epilepsy which she recalled was not particularly well controlled. Clinical examination was unremarkable, as was her 12-lead ECG. Echocardiogram was normal with normal right and left ventricular function and size. A cardiac rhythm strip had never been recorded during an episode. She was exercised on the treadmill to 15 minutes of a full Bruce protocol without presyncope or syncope. BP and pulse response were normal. Ectopy was noted at peak exercise.

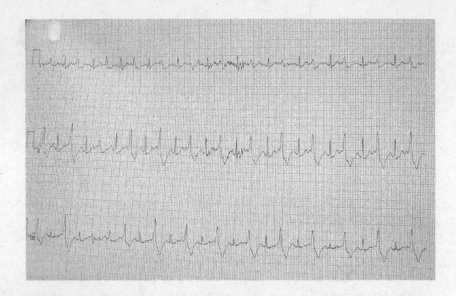

She underwent intravenous ajmaline provocation without consequence, followed later that day by adrenaline provocation. At stage 3 (of 5) although her QT interval remained normal, she developed frequent ectopy and suddenly became presyncopal, tachycardic and hypotensive. The adrenaline was stopped, intravenous β-blockers administered and within 60 seconds heart rhythm returned to normal without need for further intervention. Rhythm strips are shown below.

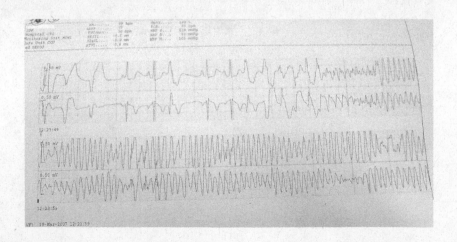

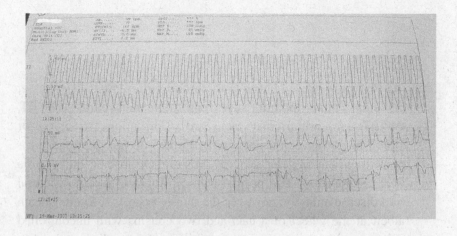

Q

Questions:

1. What is the differential diagnosis?
2. What is the rhythm that causes the hypotension?
3. What phenomenon is seen just prior to entering this rhythm?
4. What is the most likely diagnosis?
5. What treatment and management options should be given?

Answers:

1. The history suggests a tachyarrhythmia. Differential diagnosis at this stage must include supraventricular tachycardia (AVRT, AVNRT, etc), ventricular tachycardia/fibrillation (structural or normal heart ventricular tachyarrhythmias) or vasodepressor syndrome (neurocardiogenic syncope, Postural Orthostatic Tachycardia (POT) syndrome). The normal echocardiogram makes structural heart disease unlikely; however, the family history of a young death (albeit at the wheel of a car) and two cousins with uncontrolled epilepsy raise the worrying possibility of a malignant cardiac arrhythmia.
2. Initially polymorphic VT (PMVT).
3. The brief phenomenon seen pre-PMVT is bidirectional VE/VT.
4. Catecholaminergic polymorphic VT.
5. Treatment should include at least a β-blocker for life. Discussions should be conducted regarding AICD implantation and family/genetic screening.

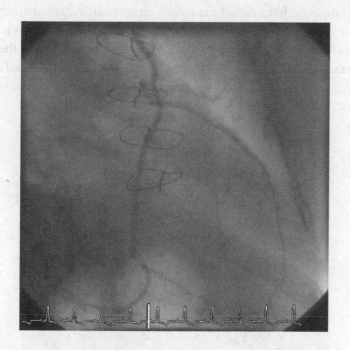

Questions:

1. What procedure has been performed here?
2. What advantages does it offer?

Answers:

1. Composite left internal mammary artery (LIMA)/radial artery coronary artery bypass graft surgery. The distal end of the LIMA has been grafted to the left anterior descending artery (LAD) and the radial artery (RADIAL) anastomosed to the side of the LIMA and then to the distal circumflex coronary artery (OMCX1/PLCX) (see below).

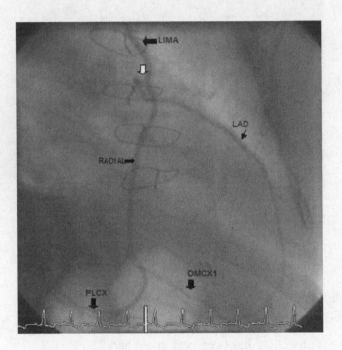

2. The advantages are that unlike conventional saphenous vein bypass graft surgery, aortic cross clamping is not necessary and use of the heart-lung machine during surgery can be avoided — offering a so-called "off-pump" surgery. It is thought that intraoperative and perioperative stroke is very uncommon, cerebral function less impaired and ITU and in-hospital stay shorter. The procedure is ideal for elderly patients with a calcified aorta and for those with previous history of stroke.

Case 51

A 20-year-old female developed palpitations when dancing in a nightclub. Although the "fluttering sensations" were initially brief, they became sustained. Her friends became concerned and called for an ambulance. Within a few minutes of the ambulance arriving, she felt faint and breathless with tightness in her chest. The paramedics recorded the ECG shown below and took her quickly to a heart emergency centre for treatment. After successful treatment, the second ECG was recorded.

First ECG:

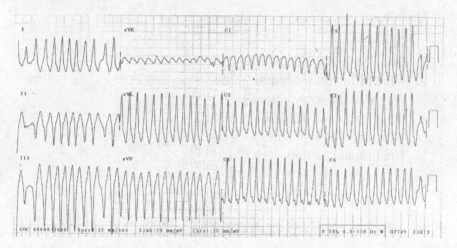

Second ECG:

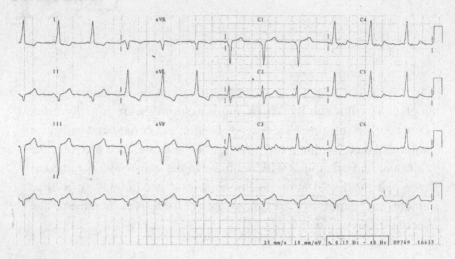

Q Questions:

1. Describe the first ECG.
2. What is the differential diagnosis of this ECG?
3. Why was she so symptomatic?
4. What treatment should be given?
5. What does the second ECG show?
6. What should be done?

Answers:

1. A broad complex tachycardia is shown, with ventricular rates approaching 300 bpm. No clear P waves are seen, and there is a notable variability in R–R intervals (200–280 ms).
2. Rapid atrial fibrillation with pre-excitation; atrial fibrillation with bundle branch block/aberrant conduction; ventricular tachycardia; antidromic atrio-ventricular re-entrant tachycardia (AVRT).
3. Low cardiac output causing hypotension as a result of a ventricular rate of almost 300 bpm.
4. DC cardioversion is the safest and most effective treatment for the shocked patient with a broad complex tachycardia. Intravenous flecainide may be used in the absence of severe hypotension (if systolic BP ≥ 100 mmHg) if the diagnosis of ventricular tachycardia is thought to be clinically excluded. Amiodarone can also be used as a therapeutic alternative but will hamper subsequent electrophysiology testing due to its long and unpredictable half life.
5. After a successful DC cardioversion, the 12-lead ECG shows Wolff–Parkinson–White syndrome, with visible δ-wave, short PR interval and wide QRS complex. The pathway can be localised to the posteroseptal/coronary sinus region using one of the several algorithms known.
6. Electrophysiological study with view to identification of the accessory pathway and its ablation by radiofrequency energy.

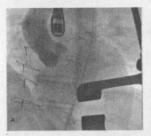
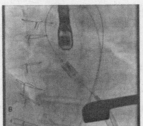
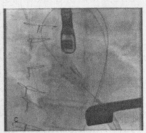

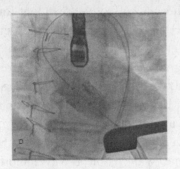
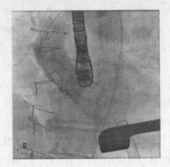

Questions:

1. What procedure is being demonstrated here?
2. What has been done in step A?
3. What has been done in step B?
4. What is happening in step C?
5. What has happened in step D?
6. What does step E show?
7. What are the indications for this procedure?

A Answers:

1. Transcutaneous aortic valve implantation.
2. Aortography.
3. The stent/valve on the balloon (between the two markers) is being positioned across the aortic valve.
4. The stent-mounted aortic valve is being deployed by its balloon.
5. The balloon is fully inflated and the stent/valve fully deployed.
6. Mild paraprosthetic aortic regurgitation is seen on aortography.
7. Severe aortic stenosis when open heart surgery contraindicated by old age or serious comorbidity such as obstructive airways disease, terminal cancer, severe cerebrovascular disease, renal/hepatic failure, or when patient refuses surgery.

This 44-year-old woman had an unexpected acute anterior myocardial infarction. Ten days later she underwent cardiac catheterisation. Left ventricular (LV) and coronary angiography were performed. The latter showed subtotal occlusion of the proximal left anterior descending (LAD) coronary artery and a long segment of severe disease in the distal half of the vessel. The LV angiogram is shown below. She underwent successful percutaneous coronary intervention with drug-eluting stents to the LAD.

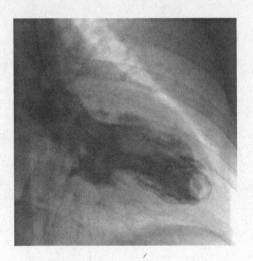

Questions:

1. What does the picture show?
2. What treatment is indicated and for how long?
3. What other medication should be prescribed?

Answers:

1. A globular apical LV thrombus.
2. Anticoagulant therapy with warfarin for a minimum of three months.
3. Aspirin for life; clopidogrel for 12 months; statin to achieve a total cholesterol of < 4 mmol/L and LDL-cholesterol < 2 mmol/L; β-blocker and ACE inhibitor.

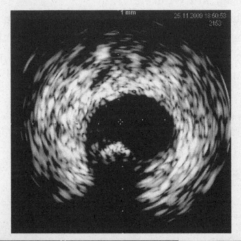

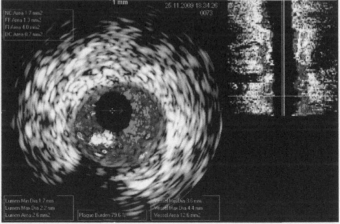

Q

Questions:

1. What are these two images?
2. What do the pictures represent?

Answers:

1. The upper image is a grey-scale intracoronary ultrasound image using the Eagle-eye® Gold intracoronary IVUS catheter and the Volcano® In-Vision imaging system. The lower image is a "virtual histology" intracoronary image of the same lesion using the Volcano VH™ software.

2. The upper image shows the central (circular) catheter artefact surrounded by dense fibrocalcific eccentric plaque in this circumflex coronary artery lesion. The bright, focal, echo-dense area at 6–7 o'clock represents calcium in the plaque.

   The lower image characterises the tissue in more detail. The red/white colours represent fibrocalcific tissue, the white colours at 6–7 o'clock dense calcium and the green/yellow colours represent fibrous plaque. The lighter green colours may indicate softer atherosclerotic plaque and even haemorrhage within it, in this patient with an acute coronary syndrome. The central (circular) catheter artefact is surrounded by the dense plaque.

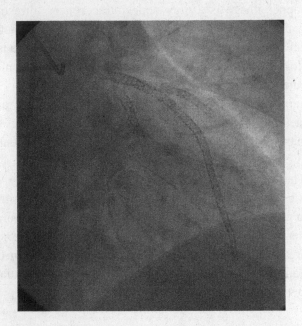

uestions:

1. What does this image show specifically?
2. What complication may be associated?

Answers:

1. This fluoroscopic image shows an extensive area of stent implantation (multiple stents in series) along the left anterior descending (LAD) coronary artery, plus further stents in the diagonal branch of LAD and in the obtuse marginal branch of the circumflex coronary artery.
2. These stents are drug-eluting stents with the intention of reducing the risk of in-stent restenosis — the commonest late complication of long areas of coronary artery stenting with bare-metal stents.

This 69-year-old lady complained of breathlessness on minimal effort over the past 12 months, with worsening hoarseness and more recently orthopnoea and ankle swelling. She had chorea as a child. Physical examination revealed a thin cachectic woman with central cyanosis and an irregular pulse. The chest X-ray is shown below.

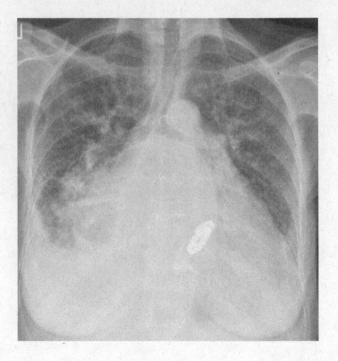

Q

Questions:

1. List nine findings on this chest X-ray.
2. What surgery has been performed?
3. What is the explanation for her clinical condition?
4. Why is she hoarse? What is the condition called?
5. What three investigations might be helpful?
6. What treatment should be considered?

Answers:

1. (i)   Mechanical aortic valve prosthesis.
   (ii) Mechanical mitral valve prosthesis.
   (iii) Tricuspid bioprosthetic valve.
   (iv) Sternal sutures.
   (v)   Gross cardiomegaly.
   (vi) Right pleural effusion.
   (vii) Splaying of the tracheal carina by a huge left atrium.
   (viii) Incorrect labelling of the "L" marker.
   (ix) Pulmonary congestion.
2. Aortic, mitral and tricuspid valve replacements.
3. She has end-stage congestive cardiac failure as a result of long-standing rheumatic heart disease, pulmonary venous and arterial hypertension, impaired right and left ventricular function. This results in anorexia, weight loss, hepatic dysfunction and skeletal muscle wasting.
4. Her hoarseness is caused by injury to the left recurrent laryngeal nerve after splaying of the tracheal carina by the giant left atrium. This condition is called Ortner's syndrome.
5. Blood count for anaemia; echocardiography; CT scan of thorax; 24-hour ECG monitoring to assess rate control.
6. Admit to hospital for bed rest, oxygen, IV frusemide, oral spirono-lactone and possibly metolazone and optimisation of heart rate control with digoxin.

A 17-year-old youth had a routine Football Association medical examination. He was found to have a systolic murmur at the second and third left intercostal spaces. The chest X-ray, echocardiogram and cardiac catheterisation data are shown below.

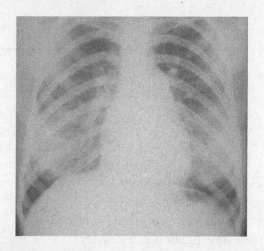

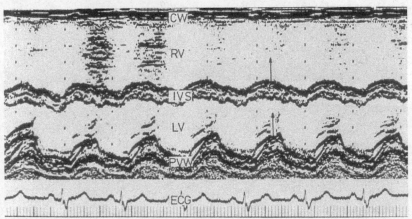

Cardiac catheterisation data

Chamber	Pressures	Oxygen saturation (%)
RA mid	mean 12 mmHg	85
RV body	45/14 mmHg	86
RV outflow		88
PA	45/26 mean 34 mmHg	88
LV	110/6 mmHg	99
Ao	112/70 mmHg	99
SVC		70
IVC		65
RA low		85
RA high		88

Questions:

1. What does the chest X-ray show?
2. What does the echocardiogram show?
3. What does the catheterisation data confirm?
4. What further investigation is necessary?
5. What treatment should be considered?

Answers:

1. Enlarged pulmonary conus and pulmonary plethora.
2. Dilated right ventricle (RV); paradoxical septal motion.
3. Step-up in oxygen saturations from SVC/IVC into the right atrium confirms atrial septal defect. There is mild pulmonary artery hypertension.
4. Two-dimensional transthoracic or transoesophageal echocardiography — to assess size and site of defect and its suitability for percutaneous closure.
5. Percutaneous or surgical closure.

A 58-year-old man presented with a three-month history of malaise, night sweats and weight loss of one stone. He complained of severe left upper quadrant abdominal pain. The appearance of his fingers is shown below. His temperature was 38.2°C; BP 160/80 mmHg; pulse rate 108 bpm. A mid-systolic click and late systolic murmur were audible with radiation to the left axilla. There was severe tenderness and guarding over the left hypochondrium. Routine urine testing showed erythrocytes and leucocytes. Haemoglobin 10.3 g/dL; white cell count 15,000/μL, C-reactive protein 150 mg/dL.

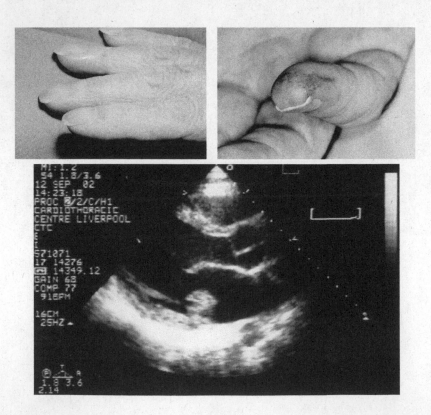

Q

Questions:

1. What questions should be asked?
2. What investigation is shown? What is demonstrated by the investigation?
3. What other tests are of paramount importance?
4. What is the likely diagnosis? What treatment is necessary?

Answers:

1. Has the patient received any dental or surgical treatment recently and did he have antibiotic prophylaxis? He had had a "wisdom tooth" removed without antibiotic cover three and one half months earlier. His parents had previously been told that he had a heart murmur but no investigations were done. His undiagnosed mitral valve prolapse/mitral regurgitation had caused no symptoms. The pictures show early finger clubbing and an Osler's node at the tip of the thumb.
2. Two-dimensional echocardiography (parasternal long axis). Large spherical vegetation is present on the posterior leaflet of the mitral valve.
3. Blood cultures and CT scan of the abdomen.
4. Infective endocarditis, with vegetation on a prolapsing mitral valve. Splenic infarction. Treatment should be commenced with intravenous antibiotics — dose and type of antibiotics dependent on results of blood cultures. Cardiac surgery is to be recommended to remove such a large vegetation and replace the infected mitral valve.

A 36-year-old electrician had noticed effort-related chest pain and breathlessness over the past six months, but he went to his general practitioner because he had collapsed on the squash court after several episodes of feeling light-headed. There was no significant past medical history. He was not on any medication and was a non-smoker. Physical examination revealed heart rate of 75 bpm; BP 140/80 mmHg and an ejection systolic murmur at the left sternal edge and over the second right intercostal space. The murmur radiated to the neck and the carotid pulse appeared to have a sharp upstroke. The important investigations are shown below.

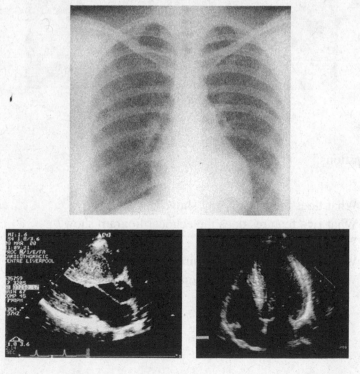

After commencing medical therapy, he underwent further treatment in the hope of reducing the recurrence of angina and syncope (see below).

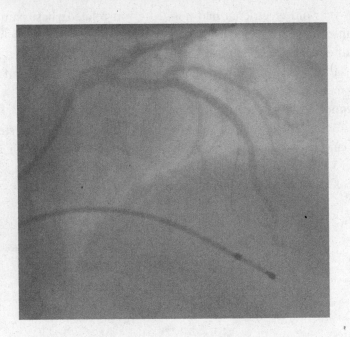

Q Questions:

1. What does the chest X-ray show?
2. What two features does the echocardiogram show?
3. What is the diagnosis?
4. What interventional procedure was performed?
5. What are three associated complications of this procedure?

Answers:

1. Cardiomegaly due to left ventricular hypertrophy.
2. Severe asymmetric septal hypertrophy and left ventricular outflow tract obstruction.
3. Hypertrophic obstructive cardiomyopathy.
4. Septal ablation using alcohol. The small inflated angioplasty balloon and the guidewire can be seen in the septal artery.
5. (i) Acute myocardial infarction and left anterior descending (LAD) coronary artery occlusion if alcohol is inadvertently injected down the LAD.
   (ii) Ventricular tachycardia/fibrillation.
   (iii) Second- or third-degree atrioventricular block. A temporary pacing electrode is shown to be placed in the apex of the right ventricle during the procedure.

This 69-year-old patient developed a persistent pyrexia and signs of a pacemaker pocket infection three months after a pacemaker generator change. He had previously undergone bioprosthetic aortic valve replacement which was complicated by intermittent second-degree heart block, requiring pacemaker implantation ten years earlier.

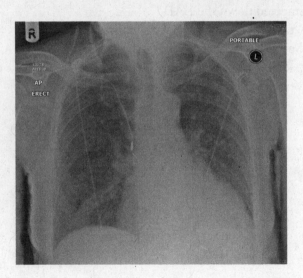

Questions:

1. What three tests should be done?
2. What procedure has been performed?
3. What complication might occur during this procedure?
4. What does the chest X-ray show?
5. What needs to be done next?

Answers:

1. Blood cultures, ECG and echocardiogram.
2. Attempted removal of the infected pacemaker system.
3. Myocardial perforation, haemopericardium and cardiac tamponade during lead extraction; tear of superior vena cava; haemothorax and pneumothorax.
4. Marked cardiomegaly. Sternal sutures. Unfortunately, the tip of the ventricular electrode has been retained in the right ventricular apex and the right atrial lead has also been retained. These passively-fixed leads can be difficult to remove but must be explanted in such a case in order to avoid septicaemia and infective endocarditis. The atrial electrode's coil structure has been partially unravelled by the applied traction before the operator abandoned the procedure.
5. The retained atrial electrode should probably be removed surgically by a cardiac surgeon although percutaneous attempts using cutting, snaring or laser sheaths might be feasible in some situations. It may be impossible to retrieve the broken tip of the right ventricular lead. Once intravenous antibiotics have controlled the staphylococcal infection, one week later, a new pacing system should be inserted via the left subclavian/left pectoral route.

This patient presented with breathlessness. His JVP was elevated and a short mid-diastolic murmur was audible at the left sternal edge. The ECG showed sinus rhythm and the chest X-ray was normal.

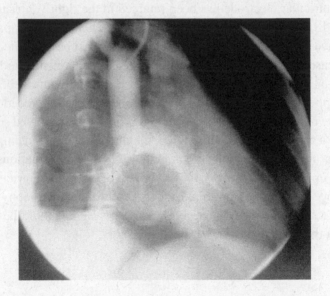

Q Questions:

1. What is this antiquated investigation? How is it performed?
2. What does it show?
3. What is the likely diagnosis?
4. What other investigation should be done that has now replaced the above?
5. What treatment is indicated?

Answers:

1. Right atrial angiogram. It is done by injecting contrast agent via a catheter into the superior vena cava.
2. Spherical mass in the right atrium.
3. Right atrial myxoma.
4. Echocardiography or gated cardiac CT/MRI.
5. The mass should be removed surgically.

This patient had a persistent pyrexia due to infective endocarditis on the aortic valve. The blood cultures grew *Staphylococcus aureus*. The temperature was 39.1°C, the white cell count 19,500/μL, haemoglobin 10.3 g/dL. The pulse (120 bpm) had a wide pulse pressure and the BP 160/50 mmHg. There was an ejection systolic murmur over the aortic area and an early diastolic murmur at the left sternal edge. The chest X-ray showed cardiomegaly and pulmonary venous congestion. On the next day, the pyrexia still persisted. The ECG showed sinus rhythm with a PR interval of 230 ms. The following day's ECG showed widening of the QRS complex and a PR interval of 278 ms. The echocardiogram is shown below.

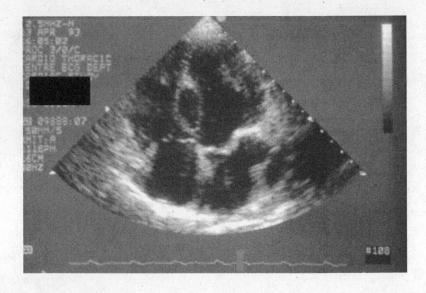

Questions:

1. What view is shown?
2. What is the diagnosis?
3. What should be done immediately?
4. What treatment is next indicated?

Answers:

1. An apical four-chamber view.
2. Interventricular septal abscess.
3. Temporary pacemaker insertion as there is a high risk of complete heart block and asystole.
4. Emergency aortic valve replacement and drainage of the septal abscess. Patching of the septum may be necessary but this is a difficult and unpredictable procedure because of the friable necrotic muscle that is present.

A 57-year-old man presented with recurrent dizziness and palpitations six years after undergoing coronary artery bypass surgery. His ECG monitor strip is shown below.

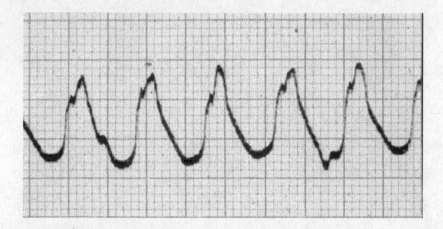

Following treatment for this dysrhythmia, he had an echocardiogram which showed severe left ventricular impairment and a large anteroapical aneurysm which was noted at the time of surgery but not resected. Subsequently, the 12-lead ECG showed sinus rhythm with anterior Q waves and a QRS duration of 150 ms.

Questions:

1. What is the diagnosis?
2. What feature on the ECG provides the evidence for the diagnosis?
3. What therapy should be recommended?

Answers:

1. Ventricular tachycardia.
2. Independent atrial activity is evident — a P wave is visible after the first and fourth QRS complex, which is clearly unrelated to the QRS complexes.
3. Therapy with an antiarrhythmic agent such as amiodarone or β-blocker should be started. An automatic implantable cardioverter defibrillator (AICD) should be offered as a secondary prevention device. This might be a resynchronisation device if either heart failure symptoms were present or if bradycardia pacing via the AICD was expected or thought to be likely.

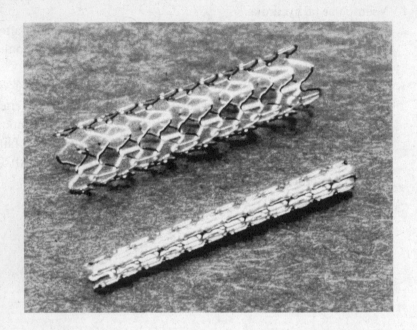

Questions:

1. What is this?
2. What is it most commonly made of?
3. What are the indications for use?
4. What advantages do they possess?

Answers:

1. A coronary artery stent — expanded and unexpanded.
2. They are generally made of high-grade stainless steel or cobalt-chromium. Stents are now designed to release certain antiproliferative drugs from the surface of their struts and future stents may no longer be made of steel but will be bioabsorbable.
3. The main indications for use are:

   (i) To optimise the acute angiographic result by preventing recoil after balloon angioplasty (PTCA).

   (ii) To prevent acute closure after PTCA.

   (iii) To treat coronary artery dissection.

   (iv) To reduce restenosis rates compared to PTCA in higher-risk lesion and patient subsets, e.g. total occlusions, diabetics.

4. Stents, particularly drug-eluting stents, reduce restenosis rates and the need for revascularisation compared to PTCA, reduce acute complications, especially acute closure, and reduce the need for emergency coronary artery bypass surgery after PTCA.

This 62-year-old man presented with unstable angina occurring over a two-week period. He had a ten-year history of hypertension and hypercholesterolaemia and smoked 15 cigarettes daily. His BMI was 32. The ECG showed small Q waves in leads II, III and AVF and T-wave inversion in V4–V6. He received aspirin, clopidogrel, atenolol, isosorbide mononitrate and statin therapy. At cardiac catheterisation, left ventriculography showed normal contractility. The coronary arteriography is shown below.

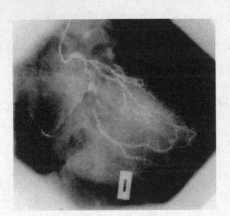 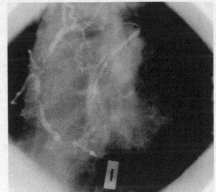

Q Questions:

1. What do the angiograms show?
2. What is the most appropriate treatment?

Answers:

1. The left frame shows narrowing of the distal left main stem, left anterior descending (LAD) artery occlusion, severe stenosis of the high obtuse marginal branch of the circumflex and an occluded circumflex coronary artery. The right frame shows occlusion of the right coronary artery and retrograde filling of the LAD via collaterals.
2. Coronary artery bypass graft surgery. His medical therapy should be optimised after surgery and lifestyle advice given.

A 65-year-old woman presented with fatigue and severe breathlessness over a four-month period, 12 months after undergoing mitral valve replacement for mixed mitral valve disease. She looked pale and possibly jaundiced. The JVP was elevated 6 cm and a soft apical pansystolic murmur was audible. There was hepatomegaly and mild bilateral ankle oedema. The chest X-ray showed cardiomegaly and marked pulmonary venous congestion while the ECG showed atrial fibrillation and right axis deviation. The haemoglobin was 7.2 g/dL; MCV 70 fL; serum LDH 3,500 IU/L; serum haptoglobin <0.1 mg/dL. Echocardiography was performed. Cardiac catheterisation showed a pulmonary artery pressure of 78/50 mmHg. A prominent V-wave was evident in the pulmonary capillary wedge pressure which was 38 mmHg (mean). Left ventricular angiography is shown below. (Left frame: diastole; right frame: systole).

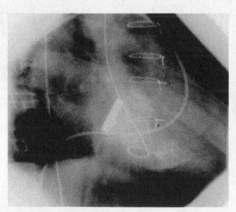 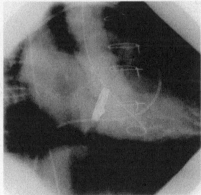

Questions:

1. What does the angiogram show?
2. Why is she anaemic?
3. What is the diagnosis?
4. What other test should be done?
5. What treatment is necessary?

Answers:

1. Mitral regurgitation.
2. She has mechanical haemolytic anaemia due to paravalvar mitral regurgitation, causing trauma to red cells.
3. Paraprosthetic mitral regurgitation.
4. Blood cultures to exclude infective endocarditis as a cause for the paraprosthetic leak; transoesophageal echocardiography to identify the exact size and extent of the dehiscense and exclude vegetations.
5. Surgical repair of the defect.

A 70-year-old woman complained of palpitations during the ECG recording shown below.

Q Questions:

1. What three features are shown on this ECG?
2. What is the likely cause of her palpitations?

Answers:

1. The ECG shows DDD pacing. Initially beats 1–8 show atrial sensed-ventricular pacing; beats 9 and 11 are ventricular ectopic beats (multifocal) causing pacing inhibition and beats 10 and 12 show AV sequential pacing.
2. Multifocal ventricular extrasystoles.

This 64-year-old man with a history of St. Vitus dance as a teenager, complained of breathlessness on effort. He was in atrial fibrillation and this was confirmed by ECG. His chest X-ray is shown below.

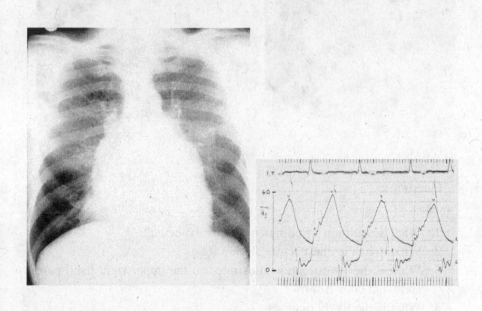

After physical examination and further investigation (above), he underwent the procedure shown below.

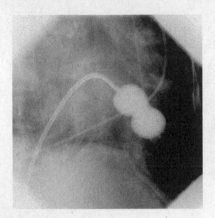 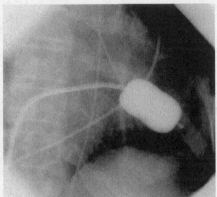

Questions:

1. What auscultatory findings might be expected?
2. What does the chest X-ray show?
3. What is the investigation illustrated in the upper right-hand panel and what does it show?
4. What is the likely diagnosis?
5. What additional investigations should be performed prior to deciding the most appropriate treatment?
6. What procedure is being illustrated in the lower two panels?
7. What features would contraindicate the technique?
8. What alternative treatment could be offered?

Answers:

1. A loud first heart sound, an opening snap and an apical, low-pitched, mid-diastolic murmur.
2. Cardiomegaly, an enlarged left atrium, pulmonary venous congestion and prominent pulmonary arteries.
3. A cardiac catheterisation trace of simultaneous left ventricular and left atrial pressures shows a mitral valve diastolic gradient of between 8–10 mmHg at rest.
4. Mitral stenosis.
5. Transthoracic and transoesophageal echocardiography and, at cardiac catheterisation, left ventricular and coronary angiography.
6. Mitral balloon valvuloplasty using the Inoue balloon.
7. Heavy mitral valve calcification; more than mild mitral regurgitation; immobile mitral valve leaflets on echocardiography/absence of opening snap; thrombus in the left atrium/appendage.
8. Mitral valve replacement.

This 57-year-old man complained of exertional dyspnoea and angina on mild to moderate effort. He gave a history of hypertension, a positive family history of ischaemic heart disease and left femoropopliteal bypass surgery in 1997. He was still smoking, was receiving treatment for hypercholesterolaemia and had a BMI of 35.1. He was on aspirin, isosorbide mononitrate, nicorandil, perindopril, atorvastatin and fenofibrate. The ECG showed sinus rhythm and left bundle branch block. Left ventricular (LV) angiography showed slightly reduced LV contractility and anterior hypokinesia. Coronary angiography showed a calcified left coronary artery with a severe stenosis above and beyond the diagonal branch (see upper left picture). The dominant right coronary artery was also calcified but there was no severe stenosis. It was decided to proceed to coronary intervention and relevant images are shown below: pre- (above left), during (upper right) and post-procedure (lower central).

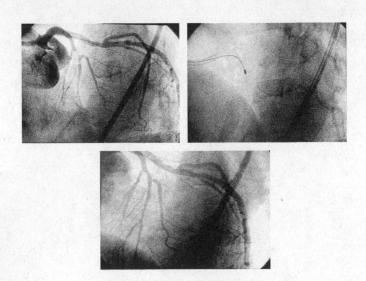

Q Questions:

1. What procedure is being performed here?
2. What are the principles of the procedure?
3. Give at least three indications for this procedure.
4. Give six contraindications.
5. What are six possible complications?

Answers:

1. High speed rotational coronary atherectomy to the left anterior descending (LAD) coronary artery, using the Rotablator® (Boston Scientific Ltd.).
2. Differential cutting — the principle of ablation of only hard material and not soft tissue.
3. (i) Calcified lesions.
   (ii) Tough, fibrotic, balloon-resistant lesions.
   (iii) Ostial lesions.
   (iv) Bifurcation lesions.
   (v) Long, diffuse segments of disease.
   (vi) Debulking prior to stent implantation.
4. (i) Contraindications to balloon angioplasty.
   (ii) Much intraluminal thrombus.
   (iii) Very distal lesions.
   (iv) Poor distal run-off especially if bulky plaque, heavily calcified lesions or large burrs are being used.
   (v) Poor LV function (< 30% ejection fraction).
   (vi) Old saphenous vein grafts.
5. (i) Coronary artery spasm (2–20%).
   (ii) Bradycardia/heart block/asystole (20–30%) — usually in right coronary or dominant left circumflex coronary arteries.
   (iii) Slow flow (2–6%).
   (iv) Coronary perforation (1%).
   (v) Cardiac enzyme (CK-MB) elevation (15%).
   (vi) Q-wave myocardial infarction (Q-MI) (1–2%).
   (vii) Death (< 1%).

This patient had an automatic implantable cardioverter defibrillator implanted using the left subclavian vein for electrode access. Shortly after completion of the procedure, she complained of breathlessness and sharp pain in the left shoulder and left upper chest, especially on coughing or breathing deeply. A chest X-ray was done and is shown below.

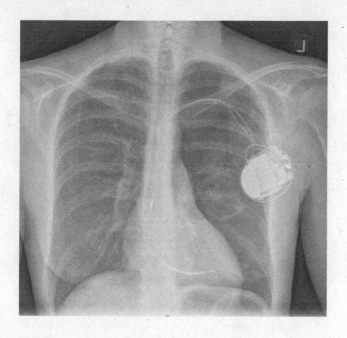

Questions:

1. What does the chest X-ray show?
2. What should be done?

Answers:

1. A left-sided pneumothorax.
2. An underwater-seal drain should be inserted in the left upper chest or in the left axilla. Smaller pneumothoraces may be treated conservatively with repeat chest X-rays and/or needle aspiration.

This 40-year-old patient had recurrent palpitations and was unresponsive to drug therapy. He underwent an electrophysiology procedure shown below.

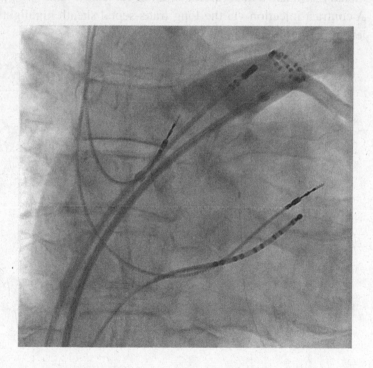

uestions:

1. There are five electrodes visible in the picture, where are they positioned and what does the contrast injection show?

Answers:

1. Actively-fixed permanent pacing electrodes are placed in the right atrial appendage and in the right ventricular septum — screwed into the septum. A decapolar electrode is positioned within the coronary sinus to record left atrial activity. A multipolar ring electrode is placed (via a trans-septal atrial puncture) in the left upper pulmonary vein and a quadripolar ablation catheter is similarly placed. A contrast injection via the long trans-septal sheath highlights the left upper pulmonary vein.

The following traces were taken both at the start (top) and the end (bottom) of the procedure. The signals are taken from the coronary sinus (blue, only two pairs are shown), the left upper pulmonary vein (green) and a mobile ablation catheter in the left atrium (white). Three surface ECGs are shown in yellow.

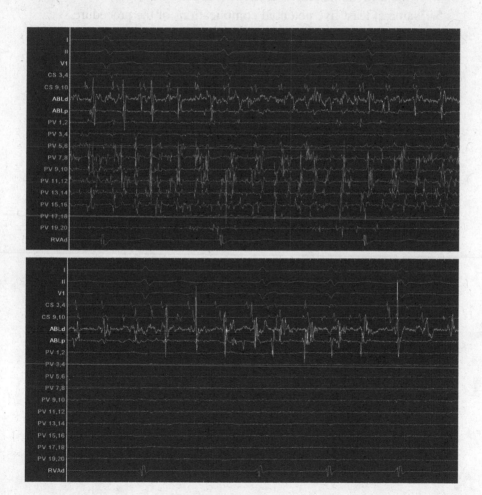

Q
Questions:

2. What procedure is being performed?
3. What do the two sets of tracings show?
4. Is the arrhythmia resolved after the second tracing?
5. Name at least five potential complications of the procedure.

Answers:

2. Pulmonary vein isolation for atrial fibrillation.
3. Irregular chaotic activity is seen in the PV ring and left atrial ablation catheters. Following successful ablation at the mouth of the pulmonary vein, no electrical activity is seen in the ring electrode, confirming electrical isolation of this vein.
4. No. Atrial fibrillation persists as can be seen by the irregular ventricular rate in the surface ECG and the persisting fast erratic activity in the ablation and coronary sinus catheters. Further ablation of the remaining pulmonary veins and potentially other left atrial sites will be required to restore sinus rhythm.
5. (i)   Cardiac tamponade/pericardial effusion.
   (ii) Pulmonary vein stenosis.
   (iii) Proarrhythmia (atrial fibrillation or atrial flutter).
   (iv) Stroke.
   (v)   Need for pacemaker.
   (vi) Existing pacemaker electrode displacement.
   (vii) Atrial-oesophageal fistula.

A 55-year-old lady presented with right-sided weakness and dysarthria lasting approximately 24 hours. She had no significant past history and was on no regular medication. Her cholesterol ratio was 3.3 and she was a non-smoker. On examination, she was tanned following a recent visit to Australia. Her blood pressure was 116/76 mmHg but her pulse was irregular. Auscultation revealed a soft ejection systolic murmur heard at the left sternal edge with no carotid radiation. Urgent CT scan suggested a small infarct in the region of the left middle cerebral artery.

Her 12-lead ECG showed atrial fibrillation and right bundle branch block.

An in-patient echocardiogram is performed and pertinent features are shown below before (top left) and during (top right and below central) injection of agitated saline contrast. Right and left heart valves appeared normal.

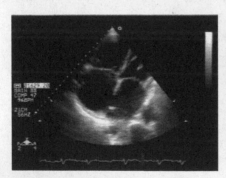 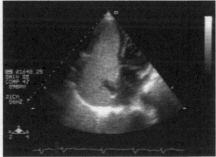

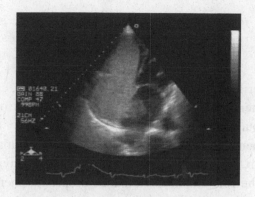

Questions:

1. What is the differential diagnosis?
2. What features are shown by the echocardiographic study?
3. What further information should be gained from the echocardiogram?
4. What further investigations should be arranged?
5. What treatment should be given?

Answers:

1. Atrial fibrillation-related thromboembolic disease, cardiomyopathy with systemic embolus, paradoxical embolus associated with an atrial septal defect (ASD).
2. Two-dimensional four-chamber view shows a markedly dilated right heart. The interatrial septum (IAS) appears hypoechoic, however in the four-chamber view the "drop out" phenomenon could explain this. A dilated right heart in the absence of pulmonary or left sided valvular disease suggests an intracardiac shunt. When agitated saline is injected intravenously, opacification of the right heart is clearly seen. A contrast filling defect on the right atrial aspect of the IAS is seen suggesting left to right flow across the atrial septum (top right), followed by clear evidence of trans-septal contrast flow from right to left atrium in diastole (lower central). A significant ASD is therefore demonstrated.
3. A shunt ratio should be obtained as well as an estimate of the diameter of the ASD. Other congenital defects should also be sought.
4. Doppler venography of the lower limbs given the recent long haul flight — to look for deep venous thrombosis. Transoesophageal echocardiography (TOE) should be performed to assess ASD size and presence of a sufficient "rim" of tissue to engage a percutaneous device.
5. Given the full resolution of symptoms together with the presence of atrial fibrillation and paradoxical embolus, anticoagulation should be commenced. This should be deferred for 1–2 weeks to reduce the risk of cerebral hemorrhagic transformation. However, aspirin should be commenced immediately. Closure of the ASD should be planned either surgically or percutaneously with an Amplatzer device depending on the findings from the TOE.

This 24-year-old woman was asymptomatic. She was referred for a cardiology opinion as she had been told that she was found to have a "cardiomyopathy" in childhood. She wondered whether she required any treatment or indeed whether any medical follow-up was necessary or worthwhile. The 2D echocardiogram and the 2D echocardiogram with colour flow are shown below.

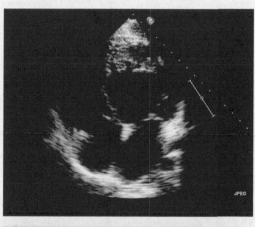

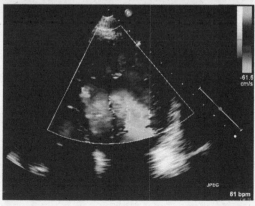

Questions:

1. What do the images show?
2. What is the diagnosis?
3. Are any other tests useful for diagnosis?
4. What are the potential complications?
5. What advice should she be given?

Answers:

1. Multiple prominent myocardial trabeculations and deep intertrabecular recesses communicating with the left ventricular cavity, as illustrated by the red-coloured, finger-like projections into the LV muscle shown on the colour flow image.
2. Left ventricular, non-compaction cardiomyopathy.
3. MRI scan.
4. Cardiac failure, tachyarrhythmias, systemic embolic events.
5. This is a congenital cardiac disorder whose clinical presentation is usually delayed into adulthood. An antiplatelet agent is probably indicated and family screening for the condition could be offered.

A 56-year-old man was admitted via the accident and emergency department. He had a long history of depression although currently was not on any medication. He presented with a 24-hour history of nausea, vomiting, abdominal pain and light-headedness. Clinically he was low in mood with a flat affect. He admitted to previous attempted drug overdoses but denied having taken any tablets. He was a gardener by trade, but business was poor. On examination his respiratory rate was 22 breaths/min, BP 100/60 mmHg with a brady-cardia of 50 bpm. Clinical examination was unremarkable apart from mild epigastric discomfort. Serum potassium was 5.4 mmol/L. Other blood tests were normal including serial troponin I, paraceta-mol and salicylate levels. Serum digoxin level was 0.2 nmol/L. Serial 12-lead ECGs are shown below.

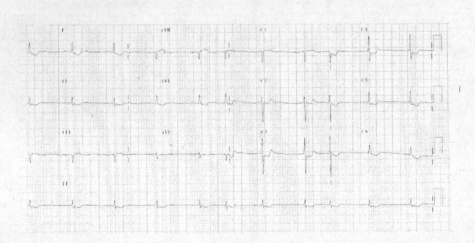

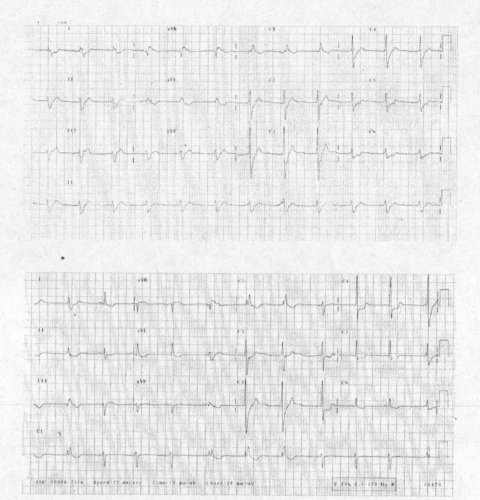

Over seven days later the symptoms and ECG abnormalities resolved without treatment.

Questions:

1. What do the ECGs show?
2. What is the likely diagnosis?
3. What is the cause?
4. What treatment options are available?

Answers:

1. The 12-lead ECGs initially showed widespread downsloping ST depression (reverse tick phenomenon) followed by varying degrees of sinus node dysfunction and intraventricular conduction delay.
2. The diagnosis is likely to be cardiac glycoside poisoning following plant ingestion. The serum digoxin level was raised indicating the ingestion of at least one of the botanically based cardiac glycosides (digitoxin, digoxin, lanatoside A, purpurea A and B, gitoxin, etc).
3. Foxglove, yellow oleander, herbal supplements and toad venom are the commonest reported such poisons. A clue may be his occupation.
4. Temporary pacing might be necessary for symptomatic bradycardia; digoxin-binding antibodies might be required if severe toxicity was evident (e.g. marked hyperkalemia due to extracellular displacement of potassium). Life-threatening arrhythmias should be treated if they arise during monitoring in the coronary care unit. Hyperkalaemia is treated in the usual way.

A 29-year-old lady presented with a long history of palpitations. She had once attended her general practitioner several years ago who after an ECG told her that she had "bundle branch block" and should really be assessed by a cardiologist. She had been syncopal twice in her adult life, but fainted on numerous occasions in childhood, usually in conjunction with fluttering in her chest. This episode was different to the rest in that it felt much more irregular and had not settled by itself.

Besides a rapid, irregular pulse, her basic observations were unremarkable and clinical examination revealed no abnormalities. The 12-lead ECG is shown below.

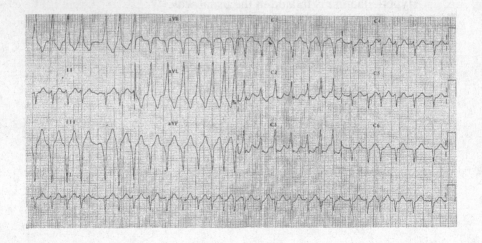

In the emergency department she was given intravenous amiodarone which changed the ECG slightly (below).

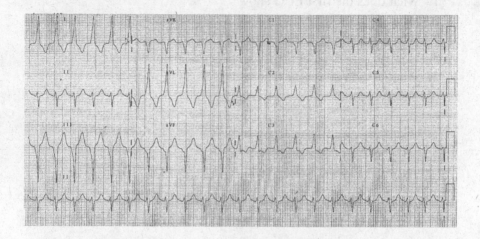

Eventually, following further amiodarone administration the heart rate slowed (see below).

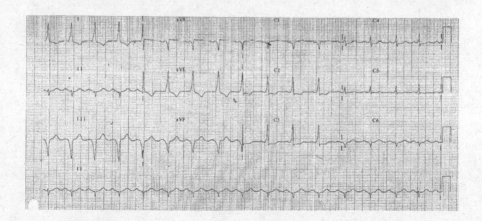

Q

Questions:

1. What does the first ECG show?
2. What does the second ECG show?
3. What does the third ECG show?
4. How do you explain the long history of palpitations/syncope?
5. What is the correct management?

Answers:

1. The initial ECG shows atrial fibrillation (AF) with a broad QRS complex and a rapid and irregular ventricular response.
2. Following the initial amiodarone bolus the atrial rhythm is regularised and slowed somewhat yet the ventricular complexes remain broad.
3. The final ECG shows reversion to sinus rhythm yet the QRS complexes remain broad. Closer inspection reveals a short PR interval and ventricular pre-excitation (see lead I) — a δ-wave, suggesting an overt accessory pathway — the Wolff–Parkinson–White syndrome. The pathway surprisingly appears not to have been affected/eliminated by the amiodarone.
4. The long-standing history of more regular palpitations probably represents atrio-ventricular re-entrant tachycardia (AVRT), whilst the most recent episode represents pre-excited AF.
5. With a history of syncope it is imperative that she is referred for electrophysiological study and pathway ablation as it is evident that the pathway can conduct at cycle lengths up to 280 ms (215 bpm) without reaching refractoriness (see shortest R–R interval remains pre-excited). Intravenous flecanide, amiodarone and/or DC cardioversion should be used as an emergency treatment.

A 21-year-old man is admitted for recurrent supraventricular tachycardia. His 12-lead ECG during sinus rhythm was normal with no evidence of a δ-wave or short PR interval. During tachycardia his QRS complexes were narrow and there were no discernable P waves.

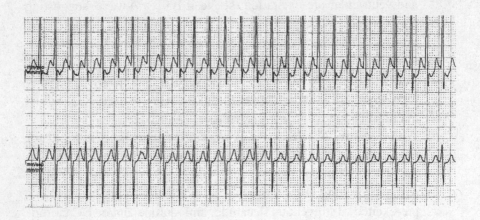

He undergoes an EP study using a 10-pole catheter in the coronary sinus (CS — blue; 9–10 proximal CS, 1–2 distal CS), a 4-pole catheter on the His (HIS — red) and a 2-pole catheter at the RV apex (RVA — orange). A selection of four surface ECG leads is shown. The first trace shows a normal sinus beat followed by a paced beat. The second trace shows the patient in tachycardia.

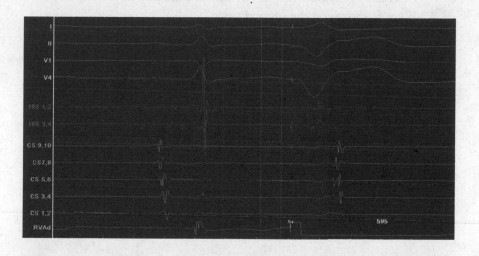

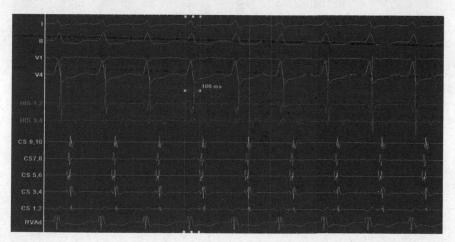

Q Questions:

1. In the first trace where is the heart being paced from? Give four identifying features of this.
2. What abnormality is shown on the first trace?
3. Explain the absence of a δ-wave on the patient's resting 12-lead ECG and describe what sort of tachycardia one might expect?
4. What is shown on the second trace?
5. What is the significance of the 100 ms green marker?
6. What is the likely diagnosis and what should be done?

Answers:

1. The single paced beat is in the RV apex. This can be seen from the "square" pulse waveform in the RVA, the "S1" (Stim) marker at the same site (yellow arrow). The earliest recorded signal after the pacing impulse being the QRS complex suggests ventricular pacing and the superior axis with left bundle morphology on the surface leads (yellow) suggests RV apex.

2. Retrograde activation from ventricle to atrium by a route other than the AV node. The earliest atrial activation seen in CS 5–6 suggests a left-sided accessory pathway as the CS catheter lies alongside the mitral annulus (see below). The normal activation of the CS in sinus rhythm (first beat) suggests a pathway that conducts in the retrograde direction only, although further pacing manoeuvres would be needed to confirm this.

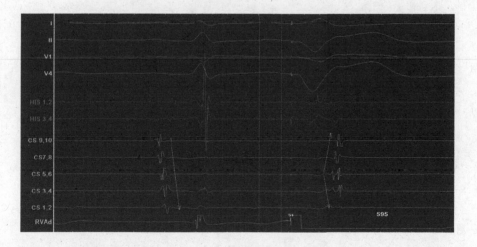

3. As stated the pathway would appear to be concealed, i.e. it only conducts in a retrograde fashion. Thus it should be able to sustain "orthodromic" AVRT with conduction retrogradely up the pathway, but it should not sustain antidromic AVRT or pre-excited AF. With no antegrade conduction, δ-waves (or ventricular pre-excitation) will not be seen.

4. The patient is in a narrow complex tachycardia with the earliest atrial activation in CS at the same site (5–6). The most common differential diagnosis of this trace alone would be either AVRT through a left-sided accessory pathway or a left atrial tachycardia with the atrial tachycardia focus occurring around the CS 5–6 site.

5. This is a measurement of the VA time in tachycardia (time from earliest ventricular to earliest atrial activation). VA times greater than 70 ms make AV re-entrant tachycardias much more likely and AV nodal re-entrant tachycardia less likely. The VA time here is 100 ms.

6. The likely diagnosis is a concealed left accessory pathway. A trans-septal puncture should be made and the pathway mapped and ablated.

A patient with an automatic implantable cardioverter defibrillator (AICD) was presented to the accident and emergency department following a series of shocks from his device. He had ischaemic LV dysfunction and underwent secondary prevention AICD implantation just over one year earlier. On admission, he was monitored in the A&E department and found to have paroxysms of a broad complex tachycardia, but he had not had a "witnessed shock". He had no chest pain, but felt unwell with tachycardia with a systolic BP of 65 mmHg. The troponin I level was normal. Two ECG rhythm strips (first two ECG strips are of one episode) are sent to the cardiologist for diagnosis and advice on further management.

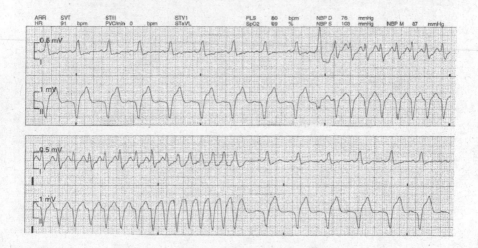

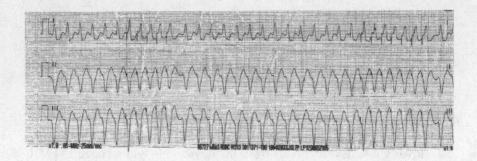

Questions:

1. What is happening with this patient and his AICD?
2. How should the patient be managed before transfer to the specialist centre?

Answers:

1. The patient is in a ventricular tachycardia (VT) storm. The first ECG shows the onset of monomorphic VT at approximately 160–170 bpm. Although it appears to be non-sustained, it is clear that the last eight beats of the VT are of a slightly different morphology to and slightly faster than the remainder of the VT. This represents a burst of antitachycardia pacing (ATP) with the clear resultant effect of termination of the VT (successful ATP). The second ECG shows the same monomorphic VT with two bursts of ATP which do not disrupt the tachycardia (failed ATP). The device will only allow a finite number of failed ATP attempts before going on to deliver the next stage of therapy — shock therapy.

2. Initially resuscitative measures should be taken. The ATP may be effective and should be allowed to attempt further therapies as required. If ATP therapies fail and the device reverts to shocks then the conscious patient should be sedated as internal cardioversion is painful. If internal shocks fail then external DC shocks should be applied when the patient is either unconscious, anaesthetised or sedated. Medical management of the VT should be concurrent with antiarrhythmic therapy (e.g. IV amiodarone, β-blockers) and potassium and magnesium supplementation. The lack of chest pain, normal troponin and presence of monomorphic VT in a patient with known severe LV dysfunction make primary ischaemia less likely but nevertheless oxygen should be applied. Once the patient is stable, he should be transferred to a specialist centre for consideration of AICD reprogramming and/or VT ablation.

Case **78**

A cardiothoracic surgical registrar requests an opinion on a 62-year-old male on the post-operative cardiac care unit. He had undergone aortic valve replacement for aortic stenosis with a 21 mm bioprosthetic valve 36 hours previously and the critical care team are having difficulties weaning his inotropic support. His mean arterial pressure is 60 mmHg and urine output between 20–30 ml/hr. He has no other co-morbidities. The surgeon says he can hear a diastolic murmur and wonders about the integrity of the aortic bioprosthesis. Continuous wave Doppler across the valve reveals a peak gradient of 33 mmHg with a mean of 15 mmHg. Pressure half time across the valve measures 600 ms. Left ventricular (LV) function is good but severe LV hypertrophy is noted.

Echocardiography is performed. Two-dimensional images are shown (parasternal long axis with aortic colour Doppler flow, aortic valve short axis with pulmonary valve and aortic valve colour flow Doppler, subcostal four chamber without colour).

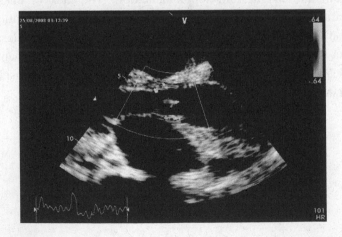

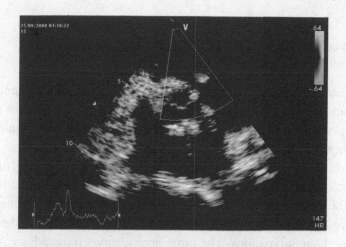

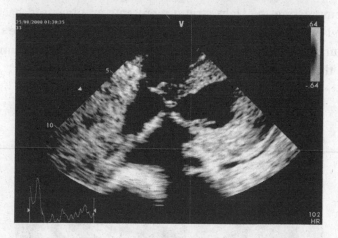

Questions:

1. What is the initial differential diagnosis?
2. Besides the information from echocardiography which is disclosed above, what four other pieces of information should be sought from the investigation?
3. What does the echocardiogram show?
4. What is the diagnosis?
5. What should be done?

Answers:

1. Cardiac tamponade, hypovolaemia/blood loss with diastolic dysfunction, sepsis. The aortic valve parameters look fine for a tissue valve (if uncertain, valve size/flow tables should be consulted).
2. Signs of pericardial effusion or tamponade; perioperative disruption of the mitral valve apparatus; right ventricular function; pulmonary artery pressure; inferior vena cava size and collapse.
3. The trivial jets of perivalvular and paravalvar aortic regurgitation are a normal post-operative finding and do not explain deteriorating haemodynamics. The large homogenous mass adjacent to and compressing the right atrium represents an organised haematoma and is likely to be producing tamponade physiology. The diastolic murmur is related to turbulent flow through the right atrium as seen in the following CW Doppler through the right atrium.

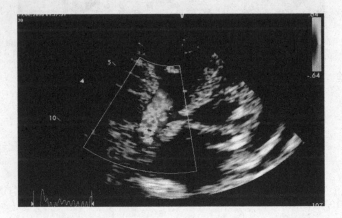

4. Cardiac tamponade.
5. Surgical evacuation. Until that can be arranged, supportive volume infusion is necessary to increase RV filling pressures. This is particularly important given the likely diastolic left ventricular dysfunction present.

A 69-year-old man presented to his general practitioner after having recurrent dizzy spells and a single blackout in his bathroom. He complained of pains and weakness in his shoulders and thighs over the past three months, which he thought was due to having had "flu" a month earlier. He had a history of hypertension and hypercholesterolaemia. He was on aspirin 75 mg daily, amlodipine 10 mg daily and simvastatin 80 mg daily. Physical examination revealed a heart rate of 45 bpm and BP 138/85 mmHg. A short, soft mid-systolic murmur was audible at the apex and he had moderate leg oedema. His blood count revealed Hb 13.2 g/dL; white cell count 9,000/μL; T4 20.1; TSH 1.3 IU/L. The resting ECG is shown below.

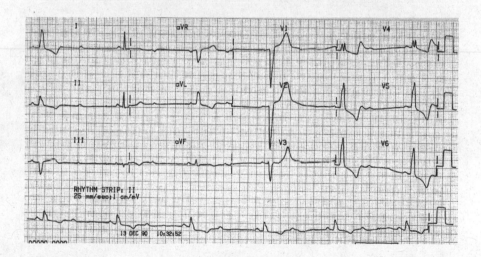

Questions:

1. What is the diagnosis?
2. What needs to be done?
3. What is the cause of his peripheral oedema?
4. What other investigations are required?
5. What else should be done?

Answers:

1. Syncope due to Mobitz Type II (second-degree) heart block.
2. Dual chamber permanent pacemaker implantation.
3. Amlodipine. This should be replaced with another antihypertensive agent. In the absence of other signs of heart failure, one might assume that the bradycardia is not a significant cause of the oedema.
4. Serum creatine kinase (CK) level. His muscle pains and weakness may be due to myositis/myopathy due to statin therapy.
5. The simvastatin should be stopped for two months, in order to see whether the myalgia/myopathy disappear. However, the symptoms may persist for more than six months in some individuals.

This 70-year-old man underwent permanent pacemaker implantation because of complete heart block causing syncope. Within a month of the procedure, he complained of recurrent dizzy episodes. He commented that the symptoms had occurred when hoeing his garden, raking leaves, lifting heavy boxes and even when hugging his wife. An ECG was recorded when repeating such an activity (see below).

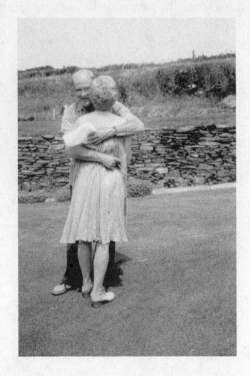

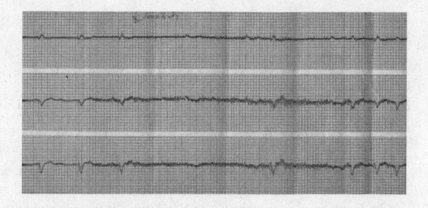

Questions:

1. What is the cause of his dizziness?
2. What does the ECG show?
3. What three things could be done to solve the problem?

Answers:

1. Myopotential inhibition of his permanent VVI pacemaker.
2. Myopotentials occur (just before the arrow) causing inhibition of pacing output.
3. There are several options:

   (i)   Reprogram to bipolar sensing if unipolar sensing is current, or
   (ii) Reduce the sensitivity of the device, or
   (iii) Reprogram the pacemaker to VOO mode if there is no underlying rhythm.

The pacemaker was reprogrammed to bipolar sensing and solved the problem. Pacing lead integrity must be checked to rule out an insulation break.

This 76-year-old man presented with a recurrence of angina 18 months after successful percutaneous coronary intervention to an occluded right coronary artery (RCA). He was still taking aspirin, clopidogrel, atorvastatin and bisoprolol since he had also undergone coronary artery bypass surgery ten years earlier. The left internal mammary artery graft to the occluded left anterior descending coronary artery was still patent as were the saphenous vein grafts to the diagonal and obtuse marginal coronary arteries. The RCA angiogram is shown below.

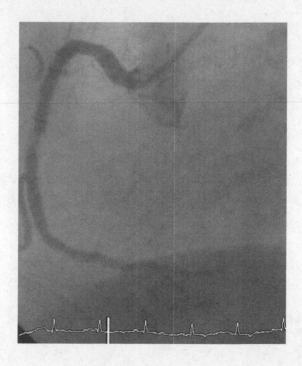

Questions:

1. What is the diagnosis?
2. What treatment is necessary?
3. How common is this phenomenon? When does it most commonly occur?
4. What factors increase the occurrence of the phenomenon?

Answers:

1. Severe in-stent restenosis within the long segment of stenting within the RCA.
2. Balloon dilatation with cutting balloon and further intracoronary stenting using a drug-eluting stent (DES).
3. 2–5% within long segments of stenting. It occurs most commonly beyond nine months with DES compared to less than six months after bare metal stenting.
4. Stenting in long segments of disease with long stents; multiple, overlapping stents; stenting to occluded segments; stenting in diabetics; small vessel stenting; stenting in saphenous vein grafts; complex stenting in bifurcation lesions.

This young woman is in the catheter lab undergoing an invasive procedure.

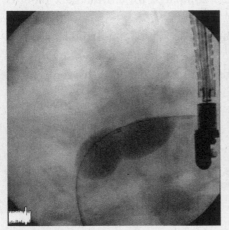 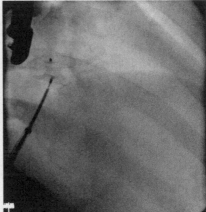

Questions:

1. What procedure is being performed?
2. What does the left-hand image show?
3. What does the right-hand image show?
4. What device is illustrated?
5. What concomitant procedure is being performed?
6. What complications may occur from the principal procedure?

Answers:

1. Percutaneous closure of atrial septal defect.
2. Sizing of the defect using a balloon.
3. Final deployment of the Amplatzer occlusion device.
4. The Amplatzer, button-shaped, occlusion device.
5. Transoesophageal echocardiography.
6. (i) Residual shunt.
   (ii) Systemic/pulmonary embolisation, e.g. transient ischaemic episode or stroke.
   (iii) Device impingement on mitral or tricuspid valves, right upper pulmonary vein, superior vena cava.
   (iv) Air embolism.
   (v) Haematoma — femoral/retroperitoneal.
   (vi) Erosion/perforation of atrial wall (rare late complication) resulting in cardiac tamponade.
   (vii) Infective endocarditis.

This 78-year-old lady presented to hospital four hours after the onset of acute anterior myocardial infarction. Her BP was 85/50 mmHg, heart rate 110 bpm. She was given aspirin 600 mg and clopidogrel 600 mg orally and taken direct to the catheter laboratory. The right coronary artery showed no significant disease and the left coronary angiogram is shown below.

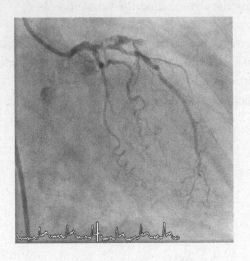

Q Questions:

1. What does the angiogram show?
2. What should the strategy be?
3. Besides emergency percutaneous coronary intervention, what additional treatment should be administered?
4. What complications might be expected?

Answers:

1. Mild narrowing of the left main coronary artery, severe ostial stenosis in the left anterior descending (LAD) coronary artery followed by intracoronary thrombus, a second severe stenosis at the origin of a septal branch and then total occlusion. There is a severe eccentric stenosis in the proximal portion of the intermediate coronary artery.

2. After intravenous/intracoronary heparin, cross the LAD occlusion with a guidewire, use a thrombectomy catheter to remove the proximal thrombus, and then open the LAD using a balloon catheter. After establishing good anterograde flow, the LAD lesions require stenting (preferably drug-eluting), from mid LAD to the origin of the left main coronary artery. Before deploying the left main/ostial LAD stent, a second guidewire should be placed into the intermediate coronary artery and its proximal lesion stented. After stenting the left main/ostial LAD lesions, the entrance into the intermediate and circumflex arteries should be opened using a guidewire and angioplasty balloon.

3. Intracoronary abciximab followed by an intravenous infusion over the next 12 hours should be administered and if no reflow or poor reflow occurs in the LAD territory, a transit catheter and intracoronary nitroprusside infusion should be considered. Intra-aortic balloon counterpulsation should be considered especially if there is any evidence of left ventricular failure.

4. No reflow, acute pulmonary oedema, hypotension, cardiogenic shock, cardiac arrhythmias and death.

This patient underwent pacemaker implantation ten years earlier because of syncope due to complete heart block. He developed recurrent dizziness over a 12-month period but could not be persuaded to re-attend hospital. Finally, he suffered loss of consciousness resulting in a fractured hip. On arrival in hospital, this chest X-ray and ECG (below) were recorded.

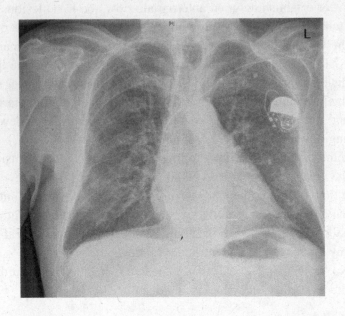

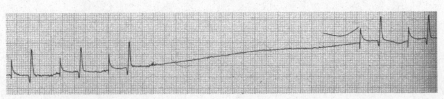

Questions:

1. What two features does the ECG show?
2. What should be done?

Answers:

1. Failure to capture and loss of output (absence of pacing spikes), i.e. at "end-of-life".
2. Emergency permanent pacemaker replacement or emergency temporary pacemaker implantation if the former cannot be arranged.

Two days after combined aortic valve replacement and coronary artery bypass surgery, this 60-year-old patient suffered repeated cardiac arrest. Over the previous 24 hours the patient had had five cardiac arrest calls for ventricular tachycardia/fibrillation (VT/VF) each responding well to a single DC cardioversion. Intravenous amiodarone (2G) was given and several boluses of lidocaine had also been tried, but the frequency of arrhythmias was increasing. The patient was being supported on adrenaline and noradrenaline with no immediate signs of being able to be weaned. He had epicardial pacing wires *in situ*. The patient's ECG between arrests showed a corrected QT interval of 480 ms. No ST-segment abnormality was noted. An echocardiogram showed only mild global LV impairment and valve function appeared normal. An ECG is found by the specialist cardiology registrar which captures one of the cardiac arrests (shown below).

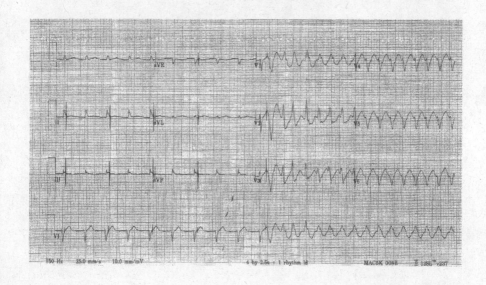

Magnified rhythm strip:

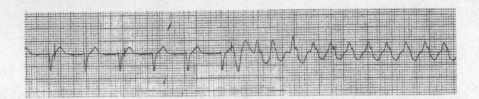

Questions:

1. What important blood tests should be sought?
2. What is the differential diagnosis of recurrent VT/VF in the post-operative setting?
3. What is the cause of the cardiac arrests in this patient?
4. What should be done to remedy this?

Answers:

1. Serum electrolytes — serum potassium, magnesium and calcium.
2. (i)   Myocardial ischaemia.
   (ii) Scar/suture-related arrhythmia.
   (iii) Severe left ventricular impairment.
   (iv) Coronary embolus.
   (v)   Electrolyte abnormalities, e.g. hypokalemia/hyperkalemia, hypomagnesaemia.
   (vi) Drug-induced long QT.
   (vii) Post-bradycardia.
   (viii) Ventricular ectopy.
   Significant QT prolongation is not present even despite the amiodarone and lidocaine. The electrolytes were normal and there was no evidence of myocardial ischaemia.
3. Pacemaker undersensing is noted with pacing spikes falling in the refractory period post-QRS complex. On the sixth visible beat (in the magnified rhythm strip) the pacing spike falls directly on the most vulnerable part of the T wave (R on T) inducing monomorphic VT.
4. The temporary pacemaker is inappropriately delivering pacing spikes due to a low sensitivity (high sensitivity value) setting. The sensing setting needs to be adjusted in accordance with the underlying R wave voltage.

This 59-year-old lady presented with sudden severe chest pain ten days after undergoing percutaneous coronary intervention and drug-eluting stent implantation to the obtuse marginal branch of the left circumflex coronary artery for unstable angina. She had been discharged on aspirin 75 mg/day, clopidogrel 75 mg/day, atenolol 50 mg/day and atorvastatin 40 mg/day. She had been smoking 30 cigarettes a day prior to her original admission. The BP was 100/60 mmHg and the heart rate 96 bpm. Her ECG showed marked ST-segment elevation in leads II, III, I, aVL, V5 and V6.

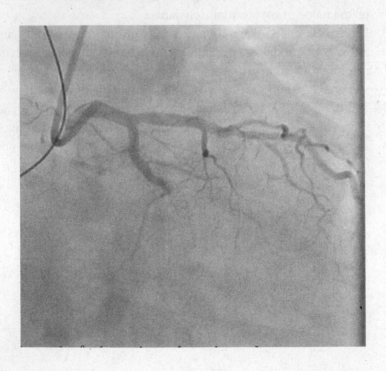

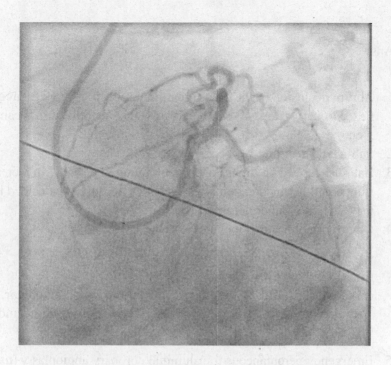

Questions:

1. What do the images show?
2. What is the diagnosis?
3. What question should be asked to the patient?
4. What are the possible causes?
5. What immediate treatment is necessary?

Answers:

1. Abrupt occlusion of the obtuse marginal branch of the left circum-flex coronary artery above the stent, whose metallic struts can be seen.
2. Sub-acute stent thrombosis.
3. Has she stopped taking the aspirin, clopidogrel or both? In fact, she stopped all her medication after discharge because she decided that they were no longer necessary!
4. Other possible causes include:

   (i)   Incomplete strut apposition/poor stent deployment.
   (ii) Clopidogrel resistance.
   (iii) Reduced efficacy of clopidogrel due to competition for the enzyme cytochrome P450-2C19 by atorvastatin and/or omeprazole.

5. Emergency percutaneous transluminal coronary angioplasty (using high balloon pressure) to the site of thrombotic occlusion and pos-sibly further stenting if necessary. Further oral aspirin 600 mg/day and clopidogrel 600 mg/day loading, intravenous heparin and intracoronary followed by intravenous abciximab. Intracoronary ultrasound might be helpful to identify poor stent strut apposition.

This 36-year-old Pakistani male had atypical chest pain. Physical examination was normal. The chest X-ray and resting ECG were normal. His echocardiogram was also normal. An exercise stress test was performed. At 1 minute 10 seconds of the Bruce protocol the ECG is shown below.

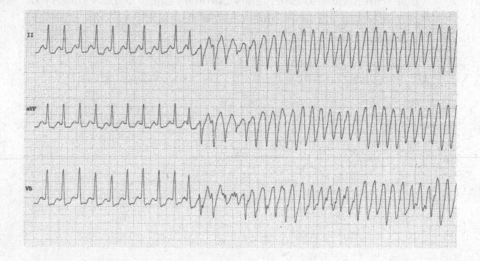

Questions:

1. What clinical event occurs?
2. What two abnormalities are illustrated on the ECG?
3. What is this called?
4. What is the diagnosis?
5. What should be done immediately?
6. What should be done next?

Answers:

1. Sudden collapse due to cardiac arrest on the treadmill.
2. Significant ST-segment depression and fast ventricular tachycardia.
3. Torsade de pointes ventricular tachycardia.
4. Severe coronary artery disease is most likely.
5. Immediate cardiopulmonary resuscitation including immediate cardioversion using the defibrillator available in the exercise room.
6. Transfer to the coronary care unit; 100% oxygen; IV heparin and glyceryl trinitrate; oral aspirin 300 mg; urgent cardiac catheterisation with a view to emergency coronary artery bypass surgery or percutaneous coronary intervention depending on the coronary anatomy.

A 70-year-old female underwent pacemaker implantation four years earlier for sinus node disease, with documented symptomatic sinus pauses. She underwent dual chamber pacemaker implantation. After three years she developed atrial flutter and was managed conservatively with anticoagulation only. Her pacemaker was switched to ·VVIR mode. You are asked to see her in pacemaker clinic due to a problem on her ventricular lead. The lead impedance is < 200 Ω in bipolar and 350 Ω in unipolar mode. The strip below is shown to you:

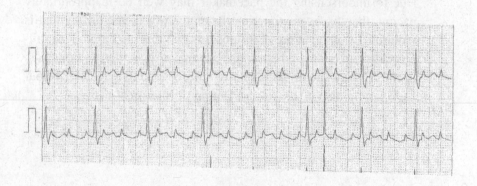

Q Questions:

1. What does the ECG show?
2. What does the impedance imply?
3. What important data should be taken from the pacemaker interrogation?
4. What investigations should be done next?

Answers:

1. Atrial flutter with a slow flutter cycle length with ventricular (V) undersensing and inappropriate pacing in the T wave. Although it appears that the pacing spike does not capture (loss of capture), this is likely to be functional due to pacing while the ventricle is refractory (i.e. unable to be stimulated).

2. The low lead impedance suggests a break in the insulation of the lead. The apparent functionality and satisfactory impedance of the pacing circuit in unipolar (i.e. using the inner lead coil only) suggests that the insulation break is only in the outer insulation at the moment.

3. The amount of V pacing should be assessed using device interrogation. Due to undersensing the pacemaker may well be inappropriately pacing, thereby overestimating the amount of actual pacing that is required. Looking at previous amounts of V pacing before lead failure will help decide whether the pacemaker is being used much.

4. A chest X-ray should be taken to look for lead damage. A 24-hour ECG would also be useful in planning further treatment.

Recent pacing histograms show 25% V pacing, but the previous 18 months' worth of clinic visits show < 1% V pacing. She is programmed to OVO and returns after one month. She has remained asymptomatic, without syncope or presyncope. A selection of her 24-hour ECG is shown below.

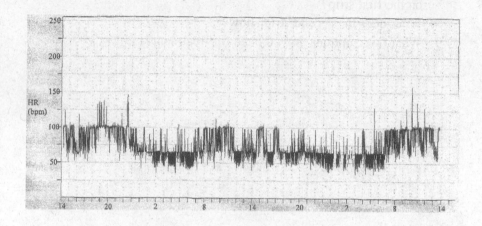

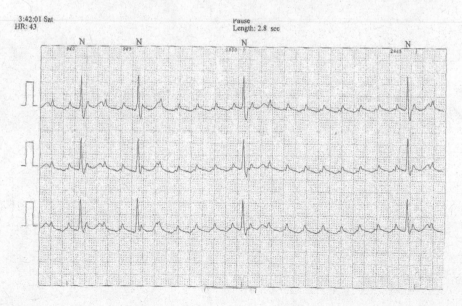

Questions:

5. What is the first strip?
6. What does it show?
7. How is the atrial flutter predominantly conducted in this lady based on the first strip?
8. What does the second strip show?
9. What three options do you have for treatment?

Answers:

5. This is a 24-hour heart rate monitor (tachogram).
6. It shows predominantly two tiers of heart rate variability. This is commonly seen in atrial flutter where ordered 2:1, 3:1 or 4:1 conduction is common. Minute heart rates seldom drop below 50 bpm.
7. Heart rates of 100 bpm in atrial flutter usually imply 3:1 conduction as the atria usually flutter at 300 bpm. In this lady however her underlying atrial cycle length is 300 ms (200 bpm), therefore V rates of 100 and 68 bpm imply 2:1 and 3:1 conduction.
8. The second strip shows a pause of 2.8 seconds due to transient higher degrees of AV block. The strip is taken at 3.42 am and likely represents an increase in nocturnal vagal tone than anything else.
9. The initial presentation with sinoatrial disease/pauses and no AV node disease with subsequent development of persistent atrial flutter means that sinus pauses should not occur now. There is an incidence of 1% per annum of significant AV block in this patient population and therefore assessment should be made focusing on this. Replacement of the ventricular lead depends on this. With normally minimal V pacing, lack of symptoms in OVO (pacing off) and higher degrees of AV block only transiently in the night, then it is likely that V pacing is not required and the patient can be simply monitored periodically.

   An alternative strategy would be to concentrate on the restoration of sinus rhythm with an atrial flutter ablation. When in sinus rhythm the Wenkebach point of the AV node could be assessed by progressive atrial pacing and if satisfactory the sinus rate could be supported in the long term using the functional (but currently switched off) atrial lead and an AAIR pacing strategy.

   A more conservative approach would be straightforward replacement of the ventricular lead although there is no hard evidence that this is currently required.

This male patient had had angina pectoris for two years, which was inadequately controlled on medical treatment. The exercise stress test produced angina and inferolateral ST-segment depression after six minutes of the Bruce protocol. The relevant coronary anatomy is shown below.

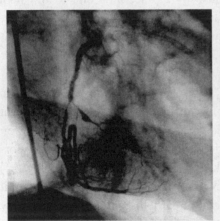
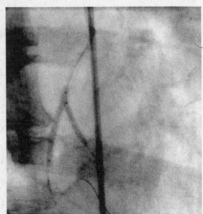
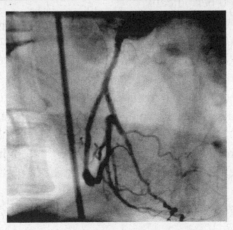

Questions:

1. What is the problem?
2. What exact procedure is being performed?
3. Apart from relief of angina, what is hoped to be improved following the procedure?
4. What late complication may occur?

Answers:

1. Severe atherosclerotic disease affecting the mid-third of the right coronary artery (RCA) and its right ventricular (RV) branch.
2. "Kissing balloon" percutaneous transluminal coronary angioplasty of the main RCA and its RV branch.
3. Hopefully, the RV function will be improved and the risks of RV infarction reduced.
4. Re-stenosis of one or both branches by fibrointimal hyperplasia.

During a cardiac catheterisation procedure, a cardiology trainee had some difficulty crossing the aortic valve in this patient although the patient had not had any documented aortic valve disease. The left ventricle-aorta "pullback" gradient was 8 mmHg. Left ventricular angiography produced the following appearance during contrast injection. Following the injection of the left coronary artery the patient became unwell, sweaty, hypotensive and developed a tachy-cardia of 120 bpm. The sequence of events on the cardiac catheter study is shown with three images of the ventriculogram and one of the left coronary artery.

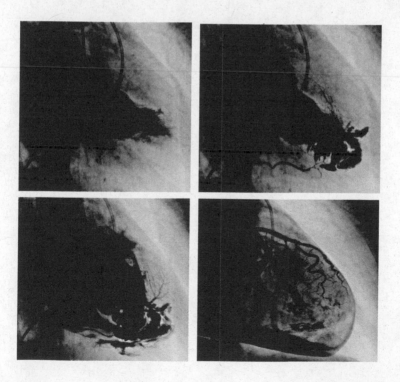

Questions:

1. What has happened?
2. What should have been done to avoid this?
3. What does the last image show?
4. What should be done immediately?
5. How should the patient be managed next?

Answers:

1. An end-hole catheter without side holes has been used to cross this aortic valve with a straight guidewire. A left ventricular angiogram was done through this catheter and with its tip directly up against the myocardium during LV contraction, a high pressure jet has been forced by the pressure injector into and through the LV wall causing myocardial perforation, haemo/contrast pericardium and cardiac tamponade.

2. (i) A catheter with side-holes and an end-hole should be used, e.g. Gensini or Multipurpose 2, or exchanged for a pigtail catheter.
   (ii) The operator should ensure that the tip of the catheter is well away from the myocardium before using a power injection for LV angiography, by using a test injection.
   (iii) The operator should stand close to the catheter so that it can be withdrawn immediately if contrast is seen to be injected into the myocardium.

3. Contrast agent is clearly seen in the pericardial space.

4. The presence of a sudden clinical deterioration suggests cardiac tamponade. This should be confirmed immediately by echocardiography and treated by pericardiocentesis.

5. Assuming the patient and the haemodynamics improve, the patient should be transferred to the coronary care unit for close observation of heart rate, blood pressure and volume of blood appearing in the drainage bag. The cardiothoracic surgical team should be informed, any anticoagulation should be reversed and blood should be cross-matched. Although the situation is very serious, catheter-related perforation of the myocardium usually settles with conservative management after successful pericardiocentesis.

This 57-year-old man complained of bloody sputum. He had twice undergone coronary artery bypass surgery 18 years and eight years earlier. He had also undergone multiple percutaneous coronary intervention procedures to saphenous vein graft disease and was currently having mild angina pectoris on medication. His medication included aspirin 75 mg/day, atenolol 50 mg/day, nifedipine retard 20 mg/day and simvastatin 20 mg/day. There were no abnormalities on physical examination except for this appearance in the mouth.

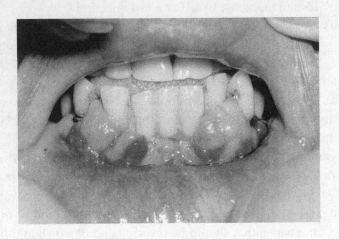

Questions:

1. What is this condition?
2. What is the likely cause?
3. What other causes are there?
4. What treatment is required?

Answers:

1. Gingival hyperplasia/hypertrophy.
2. Nifedipine.
3. (i)   Other calcium antagonists, e.g. amlodipine, diltiazem, verapamil.
   (ii) Phenytoin, phenobarbitone, cyclosporine.
   (iii) Dental caries.
4. Cessation of nifedipine and improve dental hygiene.

A 47-year-old man presented with acute shortness of breath. Physical examination revealed "a loud murmur over the praecordium" and clinical features of pulmonary oedema. His chest X-ray is shown below. He underwent cardiac catheterisation and the relevant recordings are also shown.

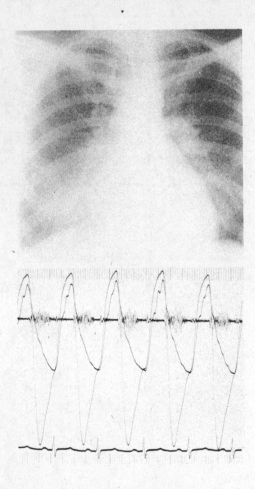

Questions:

1. What does the chest X-ray show?
2. What information is being provided on the tracing shown?
3. What does the haemodynamic data show?
4. Describe the type of murmur that is audible.
5. What is the diagnosis?
6. Name two causes for this condition.

Answers:

1. Enlarged cardiac silhouette, pulmonary oedema.
2. ECG, phonocardiogram, simultaneous left ventricular and aortic pressure traces.
3. The pressure tracings show that there is steep elevation in the LV pressure during diastole with marked increase in the LV end-diastolic pressure and equalisation of the LV and aortic pressure at end diastole.
4. The phonocardiogram recording shows a decrescendo, early diastolic murmur that occurs immediately after aortic valve closure, followed by a harsh mid-diastolic murmur — the Austin–Flint murmur.
5. Severe aortic regurgitation.
6. (i) Destruction of the aortic valve due to acute infective endocarditis.
   (ii) Acute aortic dissection.

This 18-year-old male presented with syncope and palpitations following a two-day illness of diarrhoea and vomiting. There were no abnormal findings on physical examination. Haemoglobin 12.9 g/dL; white cell count 11,500/μL; serum sodium 133 mmol/L; potassium 3.3 mmol/L; urea 10.2 mmol/L; creatinine 110 mmol/L. The chest X-ray was normal. The ECG during an episode of palpitation and syncope whilst being monitored on the coronary care unit is shown (top). A 12-lead ECG from his brother is shown below the patient's rhythm strip.

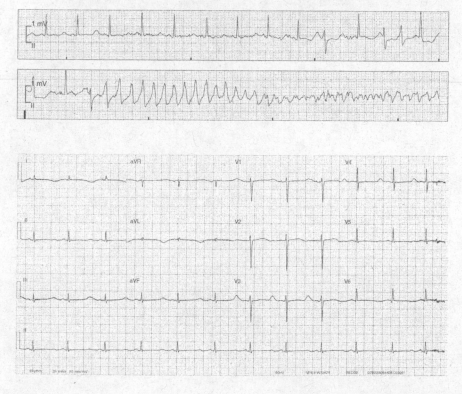

Questions:

1. What does the first ECG show?
2. What does the second ECG show?
3. What is the cause of the problem?
4. What other test should be done?
5. How should the patient be treated? What treatment would you advise for his brother?

Answers:

1. Sinus rhythm with a prolonged QT interval. Ventricular ectopic beats, R-on-T ventricular ectopic resulting in Torsade de pointes ventricular tachycardia and degenerating into ventricular fibrillation.
2. QT-prolongation (> 600 ms absolute).
3. Hypokalaemia due to the diarrhoea and vomiting has almost certainly decompensated an inherited long QT syndrome. A potassium of 3.3 mmol/L is unlikely on its own to have prolonged the QT interval to this degree.
4. Serum magnesium level.
5. Intravenous and oral potassium to correct the hypokalaemia, β-blocker followed by elective implantation of an automatic cardioverter defibrillator (AICD). His brother should have an elective AICD implanted. The family should be screened for hereditary prolonged QT syndrome, genetic screening offered and advice given on the avoidance of QT-prolonging drugs.

This 52-year-old cardiologist complained of headaches, chest pain and blurred vision over the previous ten days. He had been previously well but had stopped playing golf four weeks ago because of exertional dyspnoea and chest discomfort. On examination, he was overweight, being 95 kg at 5′ 1″ and had a ruddy complexion. He was a non-smoker but consumed 20–24 units of alcohol per week. The BP was 240/135 mmHg and the heart rate 105 bpm. A short mid systolic murmur was audible at the left sternal edge and a fourth heart sound was detectable. His chest was clear to auscultation and abdominal examination revealed no abnormalities. There was mild bilateral ankle oedema. The appearance of one of the fundi is shown. The chest X-ray showed mild cardiomegaly but clear lung fields. His ECG is shown below.

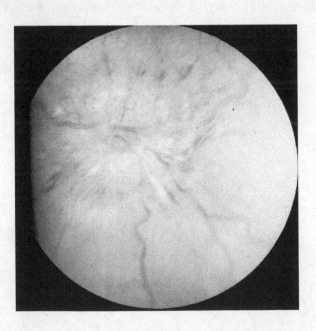

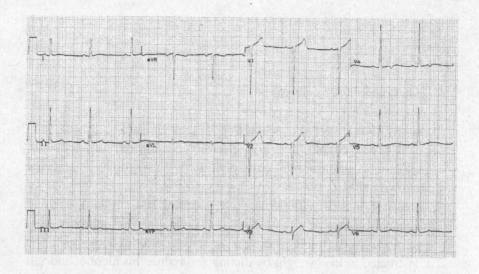

Problem ... to ... right of ... and has liver ... and ... Although ... is likely, ... and ... examination ... glass ... should ... reason ... fundus ...

Questions:

1. What is the diagnosis?
2. What abnormalities are shown by fundoscopy?
3. What does the ECG show?
4. What investigations should be organised?
5. What treatment should be initiated?

Answers:

1. Malignant hypertension.
2. Papilloedema.
3. Sinus rhythm, left ventricular hypertrophy and strain.
4. Full blood count, urea and electrolytes, 24-hour urinary cate-cholamine and protein excretion. Echocardiography and renal ultrasound/MRI.
5. Bed rest, sedation, β-blocker (e.g. atenolol 100 mg/day), calcium channel blocker (e.g. amlodipine 10 mg/day), ACE-inhibitor (e.g. ramipril 5–10 mg/day) and a thiazide diuretic. He should be instructed to lose weight by dieting and reduce his alcohol and salt intake. Although essential hypertension is likely, other secondary causes should be sought as indicated (e.g. Cushing's syndrome).

This 49-year-old man presented with severe chest pain to a district hospital and confirmed to have sustained an acute inferior myocardial infarction. He received thrombolytic therapy, aspirin, heparin and β-blocker. There was some ST-segment resolution and he remained haemodynamically stable over the next 48 hours. On the third day, he complained of feeling short of breath and nauseous. He looked anxious and sweaty. His BP had fallen to 75/50 mmHg and the heart rate had risen to 120 bpm. The JVP had become elevated to 8–10 cm above the sternal angle and a harsh pansystolic murmur was audible over the praecordium. A chest X-ray showed mild cardiomegaly and the ECG showed sinus tachycardia. An echocardiogram confirmed the diagnosis and cardiac catheterisation was arranged. Intracardiac pressures were recorded from both the right and left heart and are shown below. A right anterior oblique view (RAO) (left) and a left anterior oblique (LAO) view of the left ventricular angiogram and the right and left coronary arteriograms are shown below.

RA	20 mmHg
RV	53/21 mmHg
PA	52/35 mmHg
LV	78/10 mmHg
Ao	76/52 mmHg
PCW	9 mmHg

Oxygen saturations:

SVC	48
MPA	84
IVC	50
Left PA	84
RA	44
LV	97
RV	91
Fem A	96

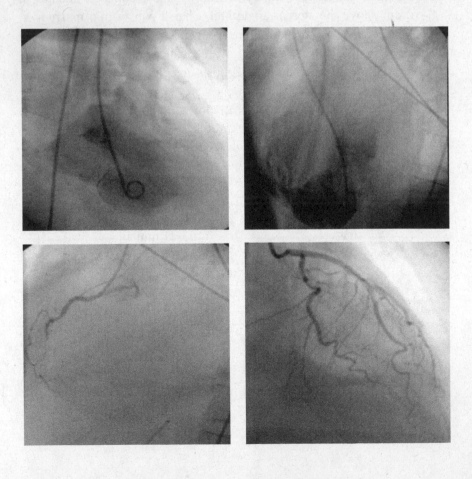

Questions:

1. What is the diagnosis?
2. What did the echocardiogram show?
3. What does the catheter data show?
4. What do the images of the left ventricular angiogram show?
5. What do the coronary arteriograms show?
6. What should be done immediately?
7. What definitive treatment should be sought?
8. What is the prognosis?

Answers:

1. Post-infarct ventricular septal defect (VSD) and probable right ventricular infarct.
2. The echocardiogram showed a large inferior-septal ventricular septal defect, right ventricular dilatation and infarction and good left ventricular (LV) function.
3. A large left-to-right shunt at right ventricular level, moderate pulmonary arterial hypertension, raised right ventricular end-diastolic and right atrial mean pressures and normal left ventricular end-diastolic and PCW pressures.

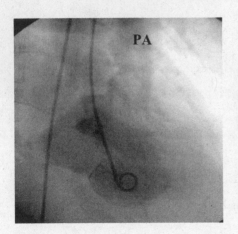 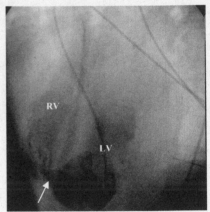

4. The RAO view shows the pulmonary artery (PA) filling during the LV angiogram. The LAO view shows a large, low ventricular septal defect (arrow) with contrast filling the right ventricle (RV) during the LV angiogram.
5. An occluded right coronary artery.
6. IV fluids to try and raise the right heart pressures and hopefully the arterial blood pressure with the aid of intra-aortic balloon counterpulsation. The latter should be inserted using fluoroscopy in the catheter laboratory.

7. Emergency cardiac surgery to repair the VSD and possibly insert a saphenous vein bypass graft into the distal right coronary artery.

8. The prognosis is not good. Despite emergency cardiac surgery to repair the defect, 30-day mortality has been reported to be up to 40%.

This 42-year-old lady gave a six week history of dull left upper chest pain and breathlessness, some of which was exercise related. There was no significant past medical history and she was not on any medication. Her mother had died from a coronary thrombosis at the age of 61 years. Physical examination was normal as was the ECG and chest X-ray. An exercise stress test was halted at two minutes because of frequent ventricular ectopic beats but there was no chest pain or significant ST-segment depression. Coronary arteriography was performed (shown below). After the third left coronary injection, she complained of feeling light-headed and short of breath with discomfort in her central chest. The BP had fallen from 120/75 mmHg to 70/50 mmHg and her heart rate had fallen to 41 bpm.

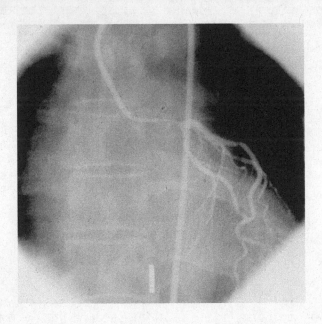

Q

Questions:

1. What is the diagnosis?
2. What has happened?
3. What four things should be done immediately?
4. What should be done next?

Answers:

1. Severe left main coronary artery stenosis.
2. She has developed global myocardial ischeamia due to left main coronary artery obstruction, possibly due to a combination of physical obstruction by the catheter whilst doing the angiogram, coronary spasm, thrombus formation or simply the vicious cycle of severe myocardial ischaemia, hypotension, poor coronary perfusion through an obstructed left coronary artery, further ischaemia, etc.
3. (i)   A bolus of 10,000 U heparin should be given via the catheter.
   (ii) Intra-arterial adrenaline.
   (iii) Cardiac arrest call, in order to secure endotracheal intubation and ventilation.
   (iv) Call for cardiac surgical team to cath lab with view to emergency cardiopulmonary bypass and coronary artery bypass surgery in the lab.
4. Emergency cardiopulmonary bypass and coronary artery bypass surgery.

Within one minute she developed ventricular fibrillation and lost consciousness. Cardioversion failed even after 100 mg of 1% lidocaine was given IV. External cardiac massage and ventilation were initiated and continued after further cardioversion was successful and replaced by sinus tachycardia with widespread ST-segment elevation seen in leads V1–V6. Without cardiac massage, the BP was only 30 mmHg.

Question:

5. What two things could be done whilst awaiting surgical rescue?

Answer:

5. A guide catheter should be inserted into the left main coronary artery using fluoroscopy. An angioplasty guidewire should then be placed into the left anterior descending coronary artery and the left main stenosis dilated with an angioplasty balloon in order to improve coronary blood flow during the cardiac massage. The guidewire should be left *in situ* until the patient is on bypass and the coronary artery bypass graft to the LAD is constructed. An intra-aortic balloon should be inserted via the contralateral femoral artery and counterpulsation commenced.

Cardiopulmonary bypass is essential in such a situation of myocardial ischaemia causing pump failure and circulatory arrest. Heroically trying to deal with the left main disease by stent implantation, although technically not too difficult to do, even in the presence of on-going external cardiac massage, will not be successful in restoring an adequate circulation to maintain a live patient. A short period on bypass and construction of satisfactory bypass grafts to the major left coronary artery branches is likely to rescue the situation by breaking the cycle described above. Such a rescue can only be offered when "on-site" cardiac surgery is available.

A 58-year-old man presented with a three-month history of exertional dyspnoea and peripheral oedema. He gave an 18-month history of watery diarrhoea. He had no chest pain and was a non-smoker. He consumed little alcohol because it caused unpleasant facial flushing. His appetite was reasonable and his weight was steady. On examination, he was normotensive and his heart and respiratory rates were normal. Cardiovascular examination revealed a raised JVP with a prominent V wave and a soft pansystolic murmur at the left sternal edge accentuated by inspiration. Pulsatile hepatomegaly was noted on examination of the abdomen. His echocardiogram and abdominal CT scan are shown below.

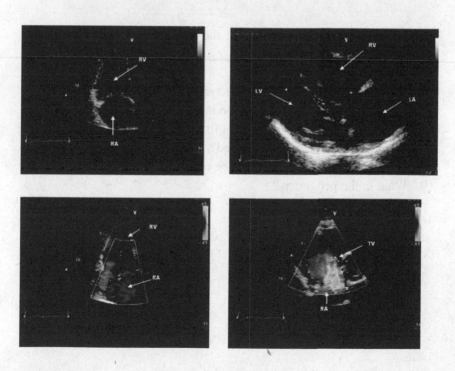

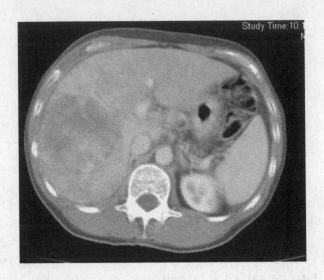

Study Time:10:

Q Questions:

1. What does the echocardiogram show?
2. What does the CT scan show?
3. What is the likely diagnosis?
4. What is the explanation for the symptoms and physical signs?
5. What three tests should be done initially?
6. How could the diagnosis be confirmed?
7. What treatment could be offered?
8. What cardiac treatment might be offered?
9. What is the prognosis?

Answers:

1. The echocardiogram shows a shortened and thickened tricuspid valve. Both the right ventricle and right atrium are grossly dilated and the cause of the dyspnoea and pedal oedema is right-sided heart failure. A moving image would demonstrate an immobile, severely regurgitant tricuspid valve accounting for the elevated JVP, prominent V wave and pulsatile liver.

2. The CT scan shows massive liver (radiolucent) metastases.

3. The diagnosis is carcinoid tumour with secondary liver metastases and associated carcinoid heart disease.

4. Carcinoid disease is a slow-growing neuroendocrine tumour commonly arising from the midgut. Approximately 60% of these tumours secrete vasoactive peptides including serotonin, bradykinin, histamine and prostaglandins. These peptides can cause secretory diarrhoea in the small bowel, fibrosis in the peritoneum, vasodilatation in the skin, bronchospasm and valvular fibrosis. The right-sided valves are more commonly affected as the peptides produced are removed in the pulmonary circulation.

5. (i) 24-hour urinary 5-hydroxyindoleacetic acid (5-HIAA) levels are increased (> 50 mg/day).

   (ii) Raised plasma Chromogranin A (CgA) levels are found in 80–100% of patients with carcinoid tumours.

   (iii) A scan with radionuclide-labeled somatostatin receptor ligand [111]Indium octreotide may identify primary or secondary carcinoid tumours (OctreoScan®).

6. Liver biopsy of the metastatic tumour will show the characteristic features of a carcinoid tumour.

7. The somatostatin analogues Sandostatin® (octreotide) and Somatuline® (lanreotide) are probably the treatments of choice for the facial flushing and diarrhoea. Arterial embolisation of the liver metastases or surgical resection may be useful to debulk the tumour and ease symptoms. The tumour/metastases do not respond well to radiotherapy or chemotherapy.

8. Diuretics and an ACE inhibitor should be considered for the symptoms of right heart failure and in situations where tricuspid regurgitation is severe, the right ventricular function remains good and the life expectancy is five years or more, tricuspid valve replacement might be beneficial.

9. 80% five-year survival for those with liver metastases. The average survival time from start of octreotide treatment has increased to about 12 years.

This 25-year-old Indian woman had St. Vitus dance at the age of six years and again at eight years and was hospitalised for nine months on each occasion. Her parents were told that her heart had been affected by the rheumatic fever. At the age of 17 years she was diagnosed as having mitral stenosis and was treated medically with diuretics. For two years she had been dyspnoeic on effort and for nine months had developed increasingly severe ankle oedema and abdominal distension with the onset of atrial fibrillation when she was anticoagulated with warfarin. Physical examination revealed a raised jugular venous pressure, a parasternal lift, abdominal distension and hepatomegaly. She had bilateral ankle oedema. Auscultation of the heart revealed an opening snap, a mid-diastolic murmur at the left sternal edge and apex and accentuation of the pulmonary component of the second heart sound. A mid-systolic murmur was audible at the apex and appeared to radiate to the left axilla. She was clinically in atrial fibrillation and this was confirmed by ECG. The axis was +93° and downsloping ST-depression was evident in leads V3–V6. The chest X-ray is shown below. Further investigations were arranged. Relevant haemodynamic traces from the cardiac catheterisation study are also shown below.

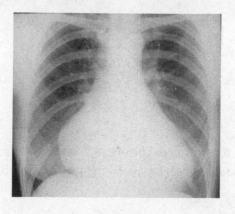

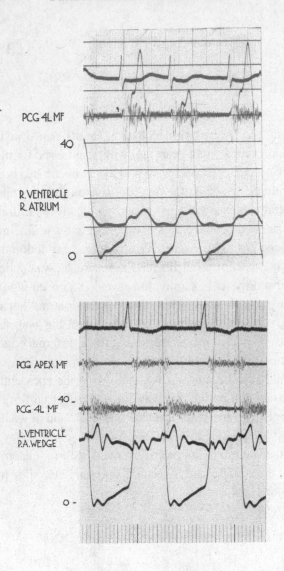

PCG 4L MF

40

R. VENTRICLE
R. ATRIUM

O

PCG APEX MF

40
PCG 4L MF

L.VENTRICLE
P.A.WEDGE

O

Questions:

1. What four features does the chest X-ray show?
2. What is the diagnosis based on the physical signs, ECG and chest X-ray?

3. What other important investigation was helpful in clarifying the diagnosis?
4. What does the first catheter trace show?
5. What does the second catheter trace show?
6. What three other tests should be done in the catheter lab?
7. What two treatments could be offered?

Answers:

1. (i)   Cardiomegaly.
   (ii) An enlarged right atrium.
   (iii) An enlarged right ventricle.
   (iv) A straight left heart border.
2. Significant mitral stenosis +/− regurgitation; tricuspid stenosis +/− regurgitation; pulmonary arterial hypertension and right ventricular hypertrophy.
3. Echocardiography.
4. Significant tricuspid stenosis with a tricuspid end-diastolic gradient of up to 10 mmHg. The right ventricular systolic pressure is between 60–80 mmHg, signifying moderately severe pulmonary arterial hypertension.
5. Significant mitral stenosis with an end-diastolic gradient between the LV end-diastolic pressure and the pulmonary capillary wedge pressure of approximately 20 mmHg. A loud mid-diastolic murmur is documented at the fourth left intercostal space.
6. (i)   An assessment of the gradient across the aortic valve.
   (ii) Left ventricular angiography.
   (iii) Aortography.

   In fact, there was no aortic valve gradient, no aortic regurgitation on aortography and only minimal mitral regurgitation on left ventricular angiography. The echocardiogram suggested mild tricuspid regurgitation.
7. Balloon commisurotomy of the tricuspid and mitral valves or open heart surgery for tricuspid and mitral valvotomy/replacement.

This previously fit 76-year-old man had fainted on the golf course. He recovered rapidly. He had always exercised regularly in a gymnasium and cycled twenty miles per week with cycling enthusiasts. A month later he reported the syncopal episode to his general practitioner when attending for a "well-man" clinic invitation. He was referred to the local district general hospital for an ECG which was reported as normal. The general practitioner requested a 24-hour period of Holter ECG monitoring and an "abnormality" was reported (shown below).

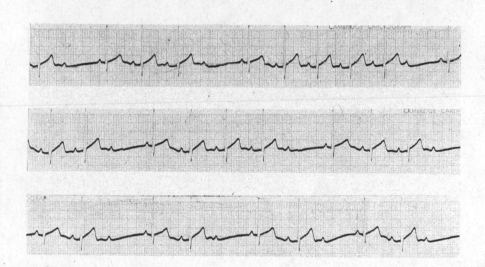

Questions:

1. What was the syncopal episode due to?
2. What does the ECG show?
3. What specific treatment should be recommended?
4. What practical reasons should be stated for making such a recommendation?

Answers:

1. A Stokes–Adams attack — probably due to transient second- or third-degree atrioventricular block.
2. Sinus rhythm and Wenkebach second degree atrioventricular block (Mobitz Type I).
3. Permanent dual chamber pacemaker implantation. Wenkebach heart block can sometimes be found in very fit, athletic individuals with a high resting vagal tone and in normal individuals nocturnally; but in this patient, the syncopal episode must be presumed to be due to a brief episode of more prolonged AV block and permanent pacemaker implantation should be recommended.
4. The patient should be told that without pacing he would probably be susceptible to further syncopal episodes which might result in injury to himself or others. Moreover, he would not be able to drive or cycle and would almost certainly have difficulty getting holiday insurance, etc.

This 60-year-old man had undergone coronary artery bypass surgery two years earlier. He had the left internal mammary artery (LIMA) anastomosed to the left anterior descending (LAD) artery and saphenous vein grafts placed to the right (RCA) and high first obtuse marginal (OMCX) coronary arteries. His total cholesterol level of 6.7 mmol/L went untreated because of poor compliance and he continued to smoke 15 cigarettes daily. He had developed recurrent angina from seven months following surgery, but had developed an episode of severe prolonged chest pain causing his admission to hospital. The ECG showed marked ST-segment depression in the anteroseptal leads V1–V4 and the 12-hour Troponin I was 12.6 μg/L. Because of on-going angina he was taken to the catheter lab for urgent coronary arteriography.

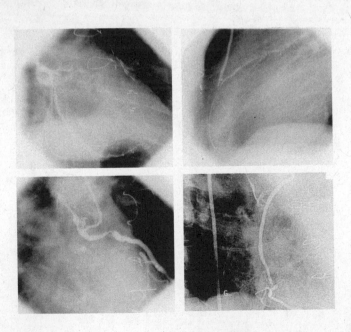

Questions:

1. What is the diagnosis on admission?
2. What do the four angiograms show?
3. Why did he develop a recurrence of angina seven months after surgery?
4. What should be done?

Answers:

1. Acute occlusion of the intermediate coronary artery causing acute myocardial infarction.
2. The top left image shows acute occlusion of the intermediate coronary artery; the top right image shows a severe stenosis of the distal anastomosis of the left internal mammary artery into the LAD; the bottom left image shows an eccentric stenosis in the body of the SVG to the OMCX, while the bottom right image shows a severe stenosis of the distal anastomosis of the RCA SVG into the distal RCA.
3. Almost certainly, this was due to the development of the distal anastomotic stenoses of the LIMA and SVGRCA.
4. Percutaneous transluminal coronary angioplasty (PTCA) and possible stent implantation to the occluded intermediate coronary artery and to the SVGOMCX stenosis. PTCA alone to the distal anastomotic lesions in the LIMA and SVGRCA may suffice. Generally, restenosis at these distal anastomotic sites is infrequent and easier to deal with than in-stent restenosis. Prior to deciding on the type of stent implantation in this man an assessment should be made of his likely level of compliance with medical therapy. He should be told that it is imperative that he stops smoking.